T0309403

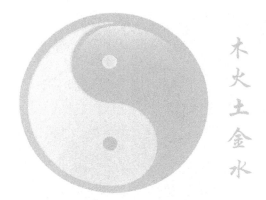

木
火
土
金
水

ACUPUNCTURE UNDERSTOOD

Rediscovering Traditional Five Element Healthcare

木火土金水

ACUPUNCTURE UNDERSTOOD
Rediscovering Traditional Five Element Healthcare

Stuart Lightbody
The Halifax Clinic of Natural Medicine, UK

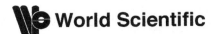

World Scientific

NEW JERSEY · LONDON · SINGAPORE · BEIJING · SHANGHAI · HONG KONG · TAIPEI · CHENNAI

Published by

World Scientific Publishing Co. Pte. Ltd.

5 Toh Tuck Link, Singapore 596224

USA office: 27 Warren Street, Suite 401-402, Hackensack, NJ 07601

UK office: 57 Shelton Street, Covent Garden, London WC2H 9HE

Library of Congress Cataloging-in-Publication Data
Lightbody, Stuart, author.
 Acupuncture understood : rediscovering traditional 5 element healthcare / by Stuart Lightbody.
  p. ; cm.
 Includes bibliographical references and index.
 ISBN 978-9814583770 (hardcover : alk. paper) -- ISBN 978-9814583787 (pbk. : alk. paper)
 I. Title.
 [DNLM: 1. Acupuncture--Popular Works. 2. Acupuncture Therapy--Popular Works. 3. Medicine,
Chinese Traditional--Popular Works. WB 369]
 RM184
 615.8'92--dc23
                                                                    2013046114

British Library Cataloguing-in-Publication Data
A catalogue record for this book is available from the British Library.

THE HALIFAX CLINIC OF NATURAL MEDICINE
22 Clare Road, Halifax HX1 2HX, West Yorkshire, England
www.naturalmedicinehalifax.co.uk

Typeset by Stallion Press
Email: enquiries@stallionpress.com

Printed in Singapore

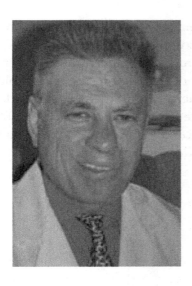

Stuart Lightbody holds a Licentiate, Bachelor and Masters qualification in Classical Acupuncture and is a member of the British Acupuncture Council. He is the acupuncture contributor for *Mens Health Matters* (Vermilion/Ebury Press), the *Hamlyn Encyclopedia of Complimentary Health* and the *Hamlyn Encyclopedia of Child Health* (Reed International Books Ltd). He has appeared on Yorkshire TV with Dr Miriam Stoppard and on Ecuadorian TV discussing acupuncture treatment and preventive medicine. He has written extensively for the *Daily Express* on preventive medicine and acupuncture and has been in practice since 1979. He is the author of *The Classic Acupuncture Points: Names, Descriptions, Functions and Locations* to be published in 2015. He is the Director of the Halifax Clinic of Natural Medicine and works in Halifax, Guiseley, York and London.

His first experience of acupuncture was in Australia in 1975 and as a result of its profound effect returned to England to attend a teaching college in Royal Leamington Spa. Over the following seven years he studied there and in the USA under Professor J R Worsley and later with the sinologist Claude Larre *SJ* of the Ricci Institute, Paris with whom he travelled and studied in China at the College of Traditional Chinese Medicine, Chengdu, Sichuan in

1984. He was a member of the teaching faculty at The College of Traditional Acupucture from 1981 until 1992.

In 1970 he co-produced a short film on river travel in northern Brazil. His account of that experience was published by the *Brazil Herald*, Rio de Janiero the following year under the title "Three Englishmen venture through Amazonia". In 1974 he studied yoga and Eastern medical philosophy at the Bihar School of Yoga, Monghyr, India under the teacher Satyananda.

Disclaimer

The reader is advised to consult their physician or qualified therapist in all matters relating to their health and particularly in respect of any symptoms which may require diagnosis or medical attention. Do not attempt to self-treat or alter your medication without consulting your doctor. The author and publisher cannot accept any responsibility for illness or injury arising out of failure to follow these guidelines.

Contents

Foreword

The man who wrote this book knows what he is talking about. How do I know that he knows? Because he has been treating me, regularly, for two decades.

I've seen Stuart when my health has been good... and when it has been not so good. When I'm feeling fine, we usually discuss the sources of potential stress in my world and how to minimise them. He'll treat me in ways which seem, somehow, to increase my ability to cope and help me turn confusion into clarity. I'll feel the better for having seen him, my energy will be on an up for many days afterwards... and the presence of a sensitive acupuncturist in my life will feel like a great supportive asset. Indeed, many a positive prediction in my regular zodiac column might not have contained quite so much optimism if it wasn't for my regular sessions with Stuart!

And when I'm not feeling so good? Well, though acupuncture does not provide a miracle cure for any physical ailment, a needle in the right spot can always lift your spirits and chase away the blues. If I've got something that requires regular, allopathic attention, I expect acupuncture to support the treatment that the conventional doctors are offering me, not to replace it!

And support it, it does, remarkably well.

Those points really work. I can feel those meridians twanging like plucked guitar strings when Stuart touches them with his needles.

Stuart's ancient Chinese predecessors knew their stuff. And he knows an impressive amount about what they knew!

If you've ever wanted to know more about acupuncture, how it works, why it works, where and when best to make it work, you're holding the right book in your hands.

Jonathan Cainer
Internationally renowned author and astrologer

Acknowledgements

My thanks go first to Professor J R Worsley who, as a renowned teacher of Five Element Acupuncture, was unparalleled in bringing alive its essence, both in the classroom and the teaching clinic. He did it with an enormous amount of humour, insight and wisdom inspiring hundreds of his students to fulfil their own personal healing potential.

To Claude Larre, SJ who brought alive the Chinese Classics for me both during a study trip to China with him in 1984 and through his co-authorship with Elizabeth Rochat de la Vallée in a series of publications called "Chinese Medicine from the Classics" (www.monkeypress.net).

To Prem Rawat who continues to remind me of the inner glory of the human being — a fact I still too easily forget.

To the following people who, through their advice, constructive comments and support have made this book a reality: Jacquie Buttriss, Jonathan Cainer, Keith Gartzen, Dr Leanne Langlois, Peter Mole (Dean of the College of Integrated Chinese Medicine), Bill Mueller, Nick Pahl (CEO of the British Acupuncture Council), Steve Paul (past director of the Centre for Psychological Therapies, Leeds Metropolitan University), and Dr David Russell.

And finally to my wife Ruth, who has been of immense support and encouragement during the writing of this book and, as a nutritionist, has helped with some of its content. This book is dedicated with love and gratitude to her and to my two children, James and Laura.

The YELLOW EMPEROR, Huang Di, asked: "I wish to be instructed on the responsibilities and functions of the 12 organs and of their relative positions in the hierarchy of the 12 Officials."

Qi Bo, the Imperial Physician, replied: "What a vast question! How can I best answer it? If you will allow me, may I ask you to follow these words:

The Heart holds the office of lord and sovereign who excels through insight, wisdom and understanding. The radiance of the spirits emanate from it. The Lungs hold the office of Minister and chancellor and are responsible for orderly and lawful conduct. The regulation of the lifegiving networks stem from it. The Liver holds the office of general of the armed forces who excels in strategic planning. Assessment of circumstances and conception of plans stem from it. The Gallbladder holds the position of an important and upright official who is responsible for what is just and exact. Determination and decision making stem from it. Tan Zhong (the Heart Protector) is like an ambassador bearing gifts of happiness and joy who guides the subjects in their pleasures. Elation and Joy emanate from it. The Spleen and Stomach are responsible for guarding the public storehouses and granaries. The Five Tastes stem from them. The Large Intestine is responsible for transit and is like the official who propagates the Right Way of Living. It generates evolution and change and the residue from transformation stems from it. The Small Intestine is like the official who is entrusted with riches and is responsible for making things thrive. Transformed substances stem from it. The Kidneys are the secretaries of labour and are responsible for the creation of power. They excel through their skill, cleverness and ability. The Triple Heater is responsible for the opening up of ditches and sluices and are in charge of the water ways. The regulation of fluids stem from it. The Bladder is like the governor of a province who is responsible for regions and cities. It stores the overflow and gathers up the fluid secretions so that they may be channelled correctly into their positions within the empire. The transformations of the qi then give out their power.

These twelve officials form an interdependent group that allows of no failing. They should do their utmost to assist one another."

"The Secret Treatise of the Spiritual Orchid" part of the **Nei Jing Su Wen Ling Shu Huang Di**. Circa 221 BCE. (Adapted from Larre and Rochat de la Vallée. p. 168.)

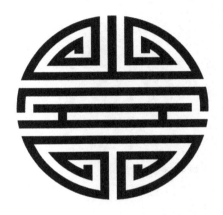

Introduction

With enough strands of DNA to encircle the Earth 700,000 times, peripheral nerve pathways of 93,000 miles in length, composed of around 10,000 trillion cells and smart enough to land a vehicle on Mars and a man on the Moon you would think this human body of ours must be the tops in the miracle stakes. But wait — there's even more to us than that. Within all of us, in the ancient Chinese view at least, lies a Kingdom with invisible energy pathways running through it. Rivers, springs, seas, mountains, stars and palaces are contained within it, all governed by an Emperor and supported by eleven Ministers.

This book goes some way in explaining this very different and enlightened view of the human being whilst, at the same time, giving advice on how this Kingdom of ours may be kept in good order.

It introduces you to the fundamental concepts of Chinese medicine, and to the different styles of acupuncture available today.

We meet some of their Emperors, learn how their palaces were built to correlate with the human body, and are given a formal introduction to each of the Five Elements in turn. Using a simple questionnaire these Elements and the way they govern our behaviour, emotions and health are described; it shows you how to recognise one that is imbalanced, and how to compensate for this by making some simple adjustments to your lifestyle. Two functions unique to Chinese Medicine, the Heart Protector and the Three Heater, both of which are unknown in Western Medicine, are described in detail (see pages 56, 57 and 68). This book gives an overview of how diagnosis and acupuncture work, what it can treat and what to expect when you first go for treatment. I also hope that it answers some of the many questions that patients ask about acupuncture, and how its renaissance today is a reflection of an accumulated wealth of experience that can be traced back to a very ancient time.

The origin of medicine in China is inseparable from the legendary Emperor Huang Di (known in the West as the Yellow Emperor) who is reputed to have lived from 2696–2598 BCE. He is considered the founder of the Chinese civilization and the one who brought together, for the first time, a systematic form of medicine. This consisted mainly of acupuncture, moxibustion, exercise, herbs and dietary advice.

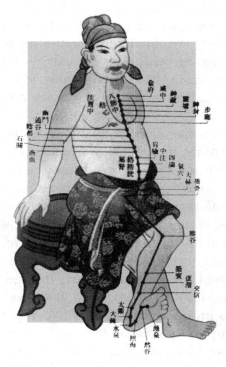

Figure 1   The Kidney Meridian

Over 2400 years later, around 221 BCE, the famous medical book *The Nei Jing Su Wen Ling Shu* or the Yellow Emperor's Classic of Internal Medicine was written. This, the world's oldest medical book in existence today, is attributed to Huang Di. Its provenance, however, is more likely to be a compilation of previous medical texts, together with information passed down orally from physician to physician, going back to this ancient time.

The *Nei Jing* is a detailed and sophisticated understanding of the energetics of the human being, of health and disease, as well as being a treatise upon life itself. What is striking is that from these ancient times has come forth a coherent and complete system of medicine that is highly effective today, both in the East as well as in the West.

One of the main factors that gave rise to the growth and refinement of this system of understanding the world around them was that of observation. The Chinese have always excelled at this. For instance, they would observe the behaviour of certain animals prior to an earthquake. Certain types of behaviour would indicate an imminent quake and thus they would be forewarned of a disaster. As an extension of this observation they built 'earthquake direction finders', the first becoming operational in 132 CE, that would point in the direction where the earthquake had taken place, so that the survivors could then be helped! In 240 BCE their astronomers first recorded the arrival of Halley's comet and by 1421 CE had charted around 1400 stars in the heavens. However, when applied to medicine, particularly the energy pathways of the body and the acupuncture points that lie upon them, this talent reached its zenith.

As these people observed phenomena that were taking place in Nature, they saw that they could all be placed in two categories; for example day and night, hot and cold, male and female, high and low, outside and inside, active and still, etc. They called these two opposing but mutually complementary aspects in Nature Yin and Yang. This theory was further developed and refined into what is now called the Law of the Five Elements.

The Fundamentals of Chinese Philosophy and Medical Theory

Dao • Qi energy • Yin Yang • The Five Elements • The Meridians

The Dao

Lying at the Heart of all Chinese philosophical thinking is a concept called the Dao (formerly the Tao). It is the unifying cosmic principle that underlies all creation in all its diversity: formless, timeless and limitless. It is from the Dao that all things spring and from which Qi energy, Yin/Yang and the Five Elements arise generating and sustaining all things in the Universe. At a more human level it also refers to the harmonious path an individual person should take on their journey through life. The originator of this concept was a semi mythical figure called Laozi (formerly Lao Tzu) who is thought to have lived around 600 BCE and who wrote the renowned Chinese classic called the *Dao De Jing* translated as The Way and Its Virtue.

Some people find the Dao a formidable concept to get their heads around, not the least because Laozi in the *Dao De Jing* says that "one who speaks of the Dao doesn't understand it; and he who does doesn't talk about it"! So right from the start it's pretty much inexplicable and unfathomable by the intellect. However, lying within each person, as it had in Laozi, is a simple feeling which only becomes apparent once the superfast mind or imagination is stilled; and it's that feeling, similarly, that can't be talked about or put into words! — it can only be felt.

Out of the Dao arose something that pervades and powers not only our bodies but the entire universe — a concept that is only just being understood by scientists who are saying that "empty space" is not a void at all but a vast, alive and vibrant cosmic web connecting all the stars and galaxies. This is because it contains an energy to which the Chinese gave the name "Qi".

Qi Energy

This vital energy is another fundamental part of Chinese culture and the basis of Traditional Acupuncture whose focus is to understand its flow, rhythms and cycles and to regulate, harmonise and enhance it within a patient. The ideogram that makes up the word "Qi" shows a pot in which rice is cooking and from which steam or vapour arises and is the Chinese way of describing it. This energy is hard to get to grips with or even see, but it is there and is the basis of life — the body's own motivating force if you like. It is made up from a number of different sources: partly from inherited energy from our parents, partly from the food and drink we consume, partly from the air we breathe and partly from emissions of electromagnetic energy in the form of solar rays and other planetary and stellar radiation. All these different energies come together to produce Qi which flows within us as a stream in a continuous cycle from our conception until the day we die. A philosopher from the Han dynasty, Wang Chong (CE 27–97) explained it another way: *"Qi produces the human body just as water becomes ice. As water freezes into ice so Qi coagulates to form the human body. When ice melts it becomes water. When a person dies he or she becomes spirit again and returns to the "great void". It is called spirit just as melted ice changes back to water"*.

To illustrate the depth of perception of the physicians of this time they further subdivided this basic Qi into a number of other categories such as Defensive (of which more is talked about in the Metal Element section), Nutritive, Ancestral, Upright, True, and Central. Another form is called Evil Qi and this is where the otherwise pure and pristine Qi has turned into something perverse or toxic often as a result of chronic unrelenting stress and conflict in a person's life. Although this is not a common phenomenon a traditional acupuncturist is trained to look out for it and to treat it accordingly so that it doesn't turn into something more serious at a later date.

Yin and Yang

From the Dao and Qi arose the idea of a duality in Nature that is termed Yin and Yang and which is another unique concept in Chinese culture and medical theory. All phenomena in the universe is viewed as consisting of varying degrees of Yin and Yang, and although they are opposites they are fundamentally complementary to one another; neither is able to exist without the other. This idea of the balance of opposites is illustrated by an early invention in China of the wheel barrow whose load sits either side of the central wheel and allows much greater weights to be carried with less strain on the arms than its European counterpart. Yang and Yin actually mean "the sunny side of the hill" and "the shady side" of it — but it's still the same hill! Crucial to this Law is that within the Yang there is always a seed of the Yin, and within the Yin there is always a presence of Yang. It's symbol is shown in the centre of Diagram 5 (p. 14). Thus, within the male resides a seed of the female, within hot there is always a degree of cold, etc. This concept is extremely simple yet most profound and can even be likened to the fundamental structure of our being in the DNA molecules' double helix configuration. A similar configuration is also illustrated in a Chinese silk painting from 2 BCE depicting two mythical figures from antiquity, Fuxi a cultural hero and Nu Wa an ancient goddess. Shown with their lower bodies intertwined they are credited with creating human kind and are the classical patrons of marriage in China.

One of the earliest references to the Yin/Yang theory is in the "I Ching" or the Book of Changes which is the oldest book in the

Yang	Yin
Male	Female
Light	Dark
Motivating	Nurturing
Waxing	Waning
Sun	Moon
Penetrative	Receptive
Heaven	Earth
Exterior	Interior
Rising	Descending
Fire	Water
Energy	Matter
Dryness	Dampness
Expanding	Contracting
Growing	Decaying

Diagram 1

Chinese culture, compiled during the reign of King Wen of the Zhou dynasty around 1120 BCE. It is itself an oracle and would be consulted in order that a pattern for future occurrences could be forecast and understood; it is still used in this way today. This Yin/Yang theory was then further developed and refined into what is now called the Law of the Five Elements.

Diagram 1 (above) is a list illustrating some of the Yin Yang complementary opposites.

Out of the interplay of Yin and Yang arise the five energetic threads, known as the Five Elements, that weave the tapestry of life, and through which the Dao as the warp thread, holds it all together.

This further extension to the Yin Yang theory bestows colour, diversity and complexity to it and allows the practitioner to under-stand and look more deeply into the patient's energetic makeup. Although there are Five Elements the Yin Yang theory still applies to them because within each Element lies both a Yin and a Yang aspect.

The Law of the Five Elements

This law is a treasure from the Oriental Medical tradition that is now just beginning to appear over our Western horizon. It is one of the most ancient ways of understanding ourselves, maintaining our health, and preventing disease. It would have begun forming in people's minds many centuries before the unification of China in 221 BCE when that country was a primarily agrarian nation. In those times the Elements or earthly materials intrinsic to nature and the Chinese way of life, were those which could sustain life and consisted of water, fire, earth, metal and wood; and to survive they needed to look after or manage these materials in an appropriate manner. Water had to be conserved so that it could support the people throughout the year, but needed to be used correctly to maintain the waterways and rice paddies and to provide fish to eat and water to drink. The forests had to be managed properly to supply wood to burn and to make utensils but trees also needed to be replanted after being cut down. Fire was needed for warmth and cooking and for smelting metals but had also to be controlled lest disasters occurred. Metal was mined and could be made into farm implements and coinage but because there wasn't much of it, and was difficult to extract, it needed to be conserved. The earth, which received the seeds and then transformed them into gifts of vegetables, grains and plants had to be left to rest, or lie fallow, for a time so that it could once again nurture growth. Thus out of this understanding came a way that mankind could sustain itself but without causing damage or wastage to the environment. Today, we would use the terms sustainability, recyling or "caring for Mother Earth", using only what we need, not falling into the trap of greed!

Most people worked in the fields at that time and consequently were governed by the effects of the seasons, the rains or lack of them, the sun, night time, daylight, their own health and strength — all influences that would give rise to the theories of Yin Yang and the Five Elements later on. As time went by they learnt to harness new

The Five Element Associations

Element	Wood	Fire	Earth	Metal	Water
Organ/ function	Liver Gallbladder	Heart Small intestine Heart Protector/ Three heater	Stomach Spleen	Lungs Colon	Bladder Kidneys
Colour	Green	Red	Yellow	White	Blue/black
Season	Spring	Summer	Late summer	Autumn	Winter
Smell	Rancid	Scorched	Fragrant	Rotten	Putrid
Taste	Sour	Bitter	Sweet	Pungent	Salty
Emotion	Anger	Joy	Worry/ sympathy	Grief	Fear
Sound	Shouting	Laughing	Singing	Weeping	Groaning
Power	Growth	Maturity	Harvest	Decrease	Storage
Direction	East	South	Central	West	North

Diagram 2

implements and machinery. These included different ploughs for different soils, new seed drills for faster planting, and the utilisation of different strains of rice that would double or even triple their food production. Much of the peasant labour was used for water control and irrigation projects which was helped by the invention of a versatile pump that could raise water over twice the height of a man, further enhancing their grain cultivation.

Furthermore these ancient Chinese observed how the movements of the planets and constellations followed a regular pattern in the heavens, and how the seasons transformed from one into another in an orderly cycle. Thus a theory was formulated incorporating the observations of these Elements in Nature which they called the Law of the Five Elements or the Five Transformations. They represent the fundamental qualities of all matter in the Universe and each have their own characteristics which, as an example, are exhibited by the different qualities of each season. The number Five is significant in Chinese culture as it is concerned primarily with order both within mankind and also in the affairs of State. There are five colours, five musical notes, five forms of punishment and five bridges leading into the Heart of the Forbidden City to name just a very few. This Law has been used to treat disease, predict the weather and divine a person's fortune as in the *I Ching*, but underlying it is an attempt to understand how life is ordered on earth and of mankind's place in it.

By the time of China's unification this theory had been further refined and allowed the physicians of that time to understand the workings of the human body. It explained how the inner energies flowed within it, how the Elements governed the functioning of the organs, how disease arose and how the Qi within could be rebalanced and regulated to return a patient to health.

In a medical text called the Huainazi, written during the second century BCE, it explains how a sage or wise person was one who is able to use the five elemental forces correctly in order to govern, rule or treat (the same word means all three in Chinese) a nation and its people. Thus we have an understanding from that time of the correct way a ruler must rule, a Minister must govern, and a medical practitioner must treat: without causing damage, loss or waste. The ruler, Minister or practitioner who could utilise these five forces or powers appropriately and effectively neither overusing nor underusing them, and who became proficient at it could then be described as a "superior person".

We all contain these Five Elements or dynamic forces of influence within us and although they are called Wood, Fire, Earth, Metal and Water they are simply labels describing the different qualities of the same energy. The Chinese term for this law is Wu Xing (meaning five steps) which indicates movement and transformation rather than a sense of them being static. These Five Elements interconnect with each other in two main ways; one nourishes and supports the next as it follows the Creative Cycle (Diagram 3, p. 12); the other keeps the forces in check in what is called the Control Cycle (Diagram 4, p. 12).

Thus in the Creative Cycle: Wood burns to create Fire, Fire produces ash which converts into Earth. Within the Earth are held the minerals and metals. Metal enriches and enables Water to exist by containing it, which in turn nourishes the trees and vegetation, the Wood Element.

In the Control Cycle: Wood is cut by Metal, Fire is extinguished by Water, Earth is penetrated by the roots of trees and vegetation; Metal is melted by Fire; Water is absorbed and contained by Earth.

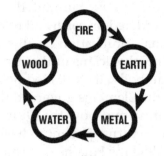

Diagram 3

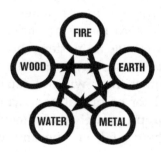

Diagram 4

The Five Elements, or energetic forces and the laws by which they function interconnect with each other in two main ways. One feeds and supports the next as it follows the creative cycle (Diagram 3, above); the other keeps the forces in check in what is called the control cycle (Diagram 4, above). Thus, in the creative cycle — Wood burns to create Fire. Fire produces ash which converts into Earth. Within the Earth are held the minerals and metals. Metal enriches and enables Water to exist by containing it, which in turn nourishes trees and vegetation — the Wood Element.

With the control cycle Wood is cut by Metal, Fire is extinguished by Water, Earth is penetrated by the roots of trees and vegetation, Metal is melted by Fire, Water is absorbed and contained by Earth.

The creative cycle is also known as the Mother/Child Law and helps us to understand how the organs and their associated energies nurture each other. Thus, using Diagram 3 (p. 12), Wood (the Gallbladder and Liver) is the Mother (the one giving nourishing qi energy) to Fire (the Heart, Small Intestine, Heart Protector, Three Heater); Fire is the Mother of Earth (Stomach and Spleen) which nourishes its children, the Lungs and Large Intestine (Metal), and so on.

The control cycle works only on the predominantly Yin organs, namely the Heart and Heart Protector (Fire) the Spleen (Earth), the Lungs (Metal), the Kidneys (Water) and the Liver (Wood). Thus, using Diagram 4 (p. 12) we can understand how the Kidney energy controls, or keeps in check the Heart, how the Heart energy controls the Lungs, how the Lungs keep the Liver in order and so on.

Today, in the 21st century, particularly in the Western cultures, acupuncture has become further refined with the emphasis on treating the patient on the emotional, mental and spiritual levels from where many illnesses arise. As you can see in the Table of the Five Element Associations (Diagrams 2 and 9, pp. 10 and 109, respectively), this theory encompasses many aspects of the human being including the organs and their associated emotions. The principal focus of the practitioner of the Five Element system is to pinpoint the one Element most in need of attention — the weak link in the energetic chain if you like. Once diagnosed and correctly supported through treatment the whole chain, that is the body, mind, and spirit of the patient is returned once more to its optimum strength and state of functioning. This holistic focus on the root imbalance is called "treating the Causative Factor" of the patient, which is commonly abbreviated to the acronym CF.

The Meridians and the 24 Hour Clock

The pathways or channels along which Qi energy flows are called Meridians. Like the energy that flows within them, they are also hard to tie down; they can't be seen and are difficult to measure but they are there and can clearly be felt during an acupuncture treatment. It was, in fact, these sensations felt within the body,

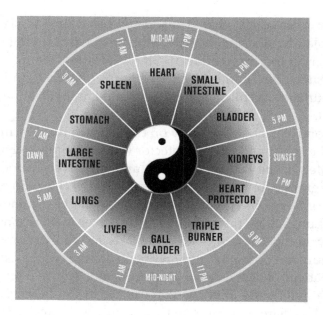

Diagram 5

observed and recorded over many centuries, combined with brilliant insights, that is thought to have led those practitioners to map out in great detail the energy pathways that flow thoughout the body.

Ask any Traditional Acupuncturist today who has been in practice for some time, and he or she will have patients who also experience these same sensations along the same pathways. Some very sensitive ones can even feel the movement of energy in the deeper pathways that connect to the inner organs themselves. This is the link between our modern times and those of ancient China. In fact the three Meridian diagrams shown in this book were drawn around 600 years ago and are virtually the same as the charts used in practice today; they illustrate the pathways of the Kidney (Figure 1, p. 2), Three Heater (Figure 2, p. 107) and the Small Intestine (Figure 3, p. 142) Meridians respectively.

There are 12 of these Meridians, whose very precise pathways traverse the body allowing the Qi energy to flow within them (see Diagram 11, p. 111). They form the very basis of all acupuncture treatment and it is through them that the exterior of the body can communicate with the interior and vice versa. In the *Nei Jing* it states *"the means whereby man is created, the means whereby disease occurs, the means whereby man is cured, whereby disease arises, the 12 Meridians are the basis of all theory and treatment"*.

The job of the Meridians is to circulate the Qi energy through our whole system, which in turn nourishes the cells and tissues and link our organs, limbs, muscles, tendons and emotions together into one complete unified organism.

As the Qi passes through each Meridian it tends to make that one meridian a little more active for the two hours that it takes to flow through it — a bit like the Severn (or Yangtse) bore but slower! Conversely, around 12 hours later the meridian is at its least active. It also follows an exact time frame beginning at 3 am GMT in the Lungs and returning to them again at 3 am GMT and flows from one meridian to another in a precise manner (see Diagram 5, p. 14).

This information is helpful in diagnosis as it gives us an idea of how our energy is at certain times of the day or night — in other words our own individual body clock. For instance, if we feel good for most of the day but very tired between 3 pm and 5 pm it can indicate an imbalance in our Water Element; if we become active and creative with our minds full of thought and ideas between 1 am and 3 am it can indicate a disturbance in our Wood Element.

Historical Background of Acupuncture and Moxibustion

Acupuncture has a very ancient tradition with a long pedigree whose origins are thought to date back to the Stone Age, a time before recorded history. Artefacts found from that era show that the needles used then were made of stone or bone and later, during the Bronze Age, of metal and bamboo. Recently, in a burial site from 113 BCE, a number of metal acupuncture needles have been discovered and, from the same era, some exquisite gold and silver ones. The use of moxibustion (the therapeutic application of heat) is thought to have predated the use of needles, particularly in the colder North of China, although they have been used together in treatment pretty much since medical records began.

In those ancient times diseases were considered to arise from the influences of evil spirits or discontented ancestors and treatment was aimed at exorcising these in one way or another. There were references to medical treatment during the Shang dynasty (c.1100 BCE) in the form of writings on "oracle bones". These were used for divination and for communication with the ancestral spirits and were the first examples of Chinese writing ever discovered. However, it really wasn't for another 900 years when the *Nei Jing* was compiled, that the beginning of an extremely well documented understanding of the body, the energy system within it, and the use of acupuncture, moxibustion and herbal medicine was marked. With the unification of China having recently taken place, medical writings began to correlate this same theme of unification to the inner workings of the human body. It was in the *Nei Jing* that the concept of an imperial power at the centre of the body with state Ministers mirroring the function of the organs first arose; its sequel is a book called the *Nan Jing* (CE 100) both of which are still essential reading for today's students of Chinese Medicine.

The earliest references to the acupuncture points are those found in manuscripts excavated from a tomb in the 1st century BCE. Some of the points mentioned in them were given names such as *Heavenly Pivot, Inner Palace, Upper Star, Spirit Hall*, and *Illuminated Sea* which are still their names in use today.

Later, in 629 CE, the first Emperor of the Tang (618 CE–906 CE) commanded that all medical knowledge in the Empire be collated and codified and it was he who founded the first major school of medicine established at this time. During the Song era (960 CE–1279 CE) more medical schools were founded and students were required to treat faculty members, government officials and military officers. Furthermore all herbal prescriptions were standardised and the Imperial Pharmacopeia listed almost 1000 items many of which were distributed inexpensively or for free during epidemics by the Imperial Pharmacy Service. In around 1026 CE the most accurate information on the acupuncture points and the meridian system was presented to the Emperor and the Chinese people in the form of a number of hollow bronze statues cast under the direction of a physician called Wang Wei Yi. These had engraved upon them the location of 657 acupuncture points together with their names. The examination system of the time, at least the knowledge of where exactly the points lay, depended upon the students being able to locate them. These statues were filled with water, covered with yellow wax, and each student was then required to needle these hidden points. This would result in a thin stream of water shooting out for the successful ones who had done their homework conscientiously! As acupuncture, moxibustion and herbal treatment became more effectively used throughout the nation, further medical books were written with perhaps the most glorious time being during the Ming dynasty.

However, with the rise in the technical superiority of Western medicine towards the end of the Qing dynasty (CE 1644–1912) particularly in treating the devastating epidemics of the time, (notably the Manchurian Plague of 1910–1911), this Traditional Medicine began to decline. By 1914 Chinese medicine was abolished and, although still widely used in outlying villages, it was driven underground during the following decades when West was considered best! However, soon after the founding of the People's Republic of China Chairman Mao, in the 1950s brought about a renaissance of Traditional Chinese Medicine and was himself treated with it during his older age which maintained his vitality into his 80's.

Nowadays, Traditional Chinese Medicine (TCM) consisting mainly of acupuncture, moxibustion, massage and herbal medicine, is commonly practised together with Western medicine throughout China. As a result its style has become ordered and standardised and is mainly focussed on the Yin Yang theory. In recent years several research institutes have been set up both in China and in Europe to further understand and develop TCM and to report on its effectiveness.

The Five Element style of Acupuncture was, and still is, considered rather too metaphysical in China for the logical and scientific principles of Marx and Mao but has been embraced in Japan, Korea, Taiwan and, particularly, the West. An additional reason for this is that the Chinese people generally steer clear of talking about the emotional side of their lives, even within their own family, because of the stigma attached to it which can affect their standing in society. Even the Emperors and their wives allowed protocol to rule their emotional lives but in this instance it was to maintain correct order for the good of the state and their dynastic line. Thus this style, whose main focus is upon the mental, emotional and spiritual aspects of the patient and from which so many symptoms arise in our western culture today, has much more acceptance in the West. The Five Element style and others, notably Japanese and Korean, tend to be more gentle and subtle and commonly uses thinner and fewer needles when compared to acupuncture practised in China.

Bringing the Chinese Medical Traditions to the West

During the 1960s some courageous and dedicated people from the West, particularly the UK, and before that, the French, who had heard of the effects of acupuncture, went out to the East to search for teachers and colleges from whom to learn. Because China was closed to foreigners at this time some went to Taiwan where many of the traditional Chinese practitioners had fled during the Cultural Revolution and others to Korea, Japan, Singapore, Hong Kong and Vietnam. These pioneers brought back their own understanding and interpretation of this system of medicine from these different countries and before long teaching establishments had sprung up in the UK and elsewhere in Europe. These colleges modified their teaching to adapt to the needs of the people in the West and the causes of their illnesses which differed from those in China and the East. Whilst these latter people suffered more from the effects of cold, damp, heat and hard physical work as well as poor nutrition the patients in the West, having pretty much overcome these sorts of external problems, were now faced with those arising from the internal ones, particularly the mental, spiritual and emotional levels. One of the amazing aspects of acupuncture is that it was, and still is, able to adapt to these different levels of disharmony whether they originate from external or internal factors, physical, mental, emotional or spiritual.

In the West patients are generally treated on a 1–1 basis rather than together in a room with ten or so other patients as in China and often the number of needles used are less, particularly those using the Five Element System.

What brought the West's attention to TCM was President Nixon's visit to China in 1972 and also an account prior to this of an American journalist being successfully treated after surgery using acupuncture and moxibustion to ease his pain.

From those days onward, the speed of assimilation into the Western culture of acupuncture, moxibustion and herbal medicine was astonishing and varied. Initially students came from North

America to study in the UK and Europe but by the 1970s and early 1980s they had established their own schools there. We now have, in the UK, well-experienced and regulated colleges which teach the traditional methods of this medical system. It is based on rigorous training both in the classroom and in the teaching clinic producing committed practitioners most of whom have to self-finance their own studies.

Around the same time sections of the orthodox medical community in the West began to take an interest in its effects. This gave rise to a more Western, theoretical approach which appealed more to the orthodox medical practitioners. However it did not attach so much importance to the historical background, the emphasis on treating the root cause, pulse taking and the holistic approach fundamental to the colleges teaching the traditional style. This has now given rise to three systems — the Traditional or Classical approach; the symptomatic approach; and one which sits in between these two which is called The Western Medical approach. The Traditional approach treats the patient holistically incorporating ancient principles and clinical observations and experiences going back over 2000 years; one uses the Western medical approach and tends to use a formulae of points. The other addresses only the patient's symptoms, again using point formulae but with much less training than the previous two.

In 1995 the five independent acupuncture organisations that existed at that time decided to unite for the greater good of the profession in the UK, and thus the British Acupuncture Council was created. This Council funds research and regulates and supports around 80% of professional acupuncturists whose members, although practising different traditional styles, do so with the same rigorous training both in the classroom and in the teaching clinic.

Different Styles of Acupuncture

There are many forms of acupuncture and have been since records began. Centuries ago, there was one school in China which focused solely on treating the digestive system of a patient and didn't bother with much else. Since then acupuncture has had its highs and lows even in China and nowadays in the West its styles have become equally varied.

There is very little regulation of Acupuncture in the UK when compared to parts of Europe and North America, even though in 2009 there were around 4 million acupuncture treatments carried out here. Pretty much anyone can practise in the UK under Common Law provided the public are safely protected. As mentioned previously there are three basic types and a number of miscellaneous ones: what divides one from the other is the length and rigour of the training process. This can vary from 3600 hours of study to as little as 30 hours and whether one addresses the whole person or just their symptoms.

The first and foremost, The Traditional or Classical Approach, relies on a detailed consultation when all aspects of the patient's life are taken into consideration with particular emphasis on their body, mind and spirit. Furthermore the observation of the patient and the taking of the 12 pulses and other traditional forms of diagnosis, distilling the practices of Traditional Medicine, are also fundamental to this approach.

This style encompasses those trained in what is termed TCM which uses the Eight Principles system of diagnosis based on the Yin/Yang theory. Another is called the Stems and Branches which utilises biorhythmic information from the day, month and year of a patient's birth date. The other is the Five Element System whose approach is covered at length in this book. Some Japanese and Korean styles, which again take a different angle, can also be included in this category. It is not as though any of these styles of Traditional Acupuncture are better than the other, as they stem from the same fundamental concepts. However, the "grid", or the method of assessing the patient's condition, and through which a diagnosis is made and, as a consequence, the choice of points and manner of treatment, is different. Each of these Traditional styles require a certain empathy from the practitioner to bring out the particular essence of that style to the fullest and in the most effective way. Some practitioners have an academic or scientific bent and are drawn to a more pragmatic style whereas others are drawn to Nature and the more esoteric view of Humankind. There are some who have the ability to combine or integrate more than one style but what unites them all is the length and rigour of the training process both in the classroom and in the teaching clinic.

The second is called Western Medical Acupuncture and is commonly practised by some western doctors and some committed physiotherapists and nurses. These practitioners are not so much interested in the historical and philosophical background of Chinese medicine, nor do they use pulse diagnosis or the traditional diagnostic observations of the patient's body, mind and spirit. They tend not to accept the existence of the meridian system nor the therapeutic benefits of moxibustion. Rather they see acupuncture as stimulating the nervous system and thus the organs and by doing so a variety of chemicals and hormones such as endorphins, are released into the system which then encourages healing and ease pain. They generally use a formulae of points together with some "trigger points", which are painful knots of muscle, and treat some of the conditions that you go to your GP for, particularly those causing pain.

The next style is called Symptomatic Acupuncture which is sometimes referred to as "Dry Needling". Here the symptoms solely are treated using, again, a formulae of points and some trigger points. This style requires very little training, perhaps a couple of weekends, and is commonly practised by physiotherapists, doctors, osteopaths, chiropractors and nurses who use it as an adjunct to their main therapy, usually for painful conditions that affect the musculo-skeletal system.

In China, even the "barefoot doctors", or "rural paramedical workers" have to complete around two years of training these days before being allowed to treat in the villages: being trained in Western medicine does not automatically mean you can competently practise the oriental version.

The following table gives the training requirements, professional bodies and contact details for these different styles.

The public are now asking why can one person set up practice after only 30 hours training whereas another can only do so after studying for 3,600 hours and then only when they have passed the

Style	Length of Training	Professional Body
Traditional or Classical	3600 hours over 3–5 years. CPD required	The British Acupuncture Council (www.acupuncture.org)
Western Medical	Approx. 80–200 hours. CPD required	The British Medical Acupuncture Society (www.medical-acupuncture.co.uk) The British Academy of Western Medical Acupuncture (www.bawma.co.uk) The Acupuncture Association of Chartered Physiotherapists (www.aacp.org.uk)
Symptomatic	Approx. 30 hours over two weekends	The British Medical Acupuncture Society (www.medical-acupuncture.co.uk) The Acupuncture Society (www.acupuncturesociety.org.uk)

CPD = Continuing Professional Development

Diagram 6

rigorous examinations. It's a good question. Whichever style you choose it is important that you enquire from the practitioner which method they use and the length of their training, both in the class-room and in the teaching clinic before you make your decision.

Miscellaneous

The following miscellaneous section covers other lesser known forms of supportive treatment some of which have an historical lineage.

Auricular Acupuncture

Also known as Ear Acupuncture this is a relatively new discovery having been developed in the 1950s both in China and in France and is based on the idea that the body and the organs are repre-sented in the ear. Some practitioners use this method as a complete system in itself but most combine it with regular acupuncture treat-ment. Although it can be used to treat a wide variety of symptoms it is often used for pain relief. It can be effective during childbirth when the points can be stimulated electronically using a TENS type machine, for drug addictions particularly tobacco, alcohol, the opi-ates and cocaine dependency and for anxiety-related conditions. Small seeds, glass beads or stainless steel ear presses, which look like a minute drawing pin, are placed on or in the ear points and are covered with surgical tape. Patients can then stimulate them to control the craving, pain or anxiety and they can be left in place for a time, occasionally a few weeks.

Electro-acupuncture and Analgesia

This style uses a machine that generates a mild electric current to stimulate the points and can be used to treat hemiplegia or one-sided paralysis following a stroke. It is also effective for pain relief. The patient can feel a mild tingling sensation or a twitching muscle during treatment. It can also reinforce treatment that requires more constant stimulation such as painful conditions and addictions. It can also be used as a form of analgesia, replacing anaesthetics for surgical operations. Although commonly used in China in this way, is not so common yet in the West. The needles, once in place, are connected to this machine and its pain-relieving effect can be controlled by the patient themselves.

Laser Acupuncture

Instead of using needles, this style utilises a thin concentrated beam of light to affect the acupuncture points. Although considered less effective than Traditional Acupuncture the advantage of this style is that it is painless and useful for those who are afraid of needles. This is still a relatively new area but there is currently research in the pipeline which will make clear which conditions this form can best treat.

Cosmetic Acupuncture

This treatment, also called Facial Rejuvenation Therapy, is one of the newest forms of acupuncture having been developed in the US in recent years. It requires some specialised training and is said to be effective in the short term for reducing facial wrinkles and improving the complexion and the facial muscle tone. It may take around 6 treatments or so for it to have a lasting effect. Very thin needles are used, mainly on the face but sometimes elsewhere which are either stimulated using a TENS-like machine or attached to pads on the skin which tighten the muscles there. Both methods often use a mild electrical stimulation. Sometimes they are manually stimulated often in conjunction with facial massage.

Cupping

Cupping has been used for centuries in cultures such as those of the Greeks, Romans and the Arab world. The cups are usually made of glass or bamboo and a vacuum is created inside the cup using a lighted taper which is then quickly placed on the skin once the taper has been removed. In this way the skin, and with it the flesh and energy, are drawn up into the cup where it is left in position for some time. The sensation is not unpleasant and is commonly used for the treatment of back, neck and joint problems, asthma and the common cold. Recently a new system has been introduced whereby the vacuum is created by pumping the air out manually once the cups have been correctly positioned.

Acupressure. Tui Na. Shiatsu

These types of treatment are in common use and take the form of massaging the acupuncture points to produce beneficial effects on the patient's energy system. Acupressure, although not as powerful as needle or moxibustion can be very effective in the short term for problems such as stiff muscles and tendons, in emergency situations and in the treatment of children. Shiatsu and Tui Na, from the Japanese and Chinese traditions respectively, use specific types of massage techniques which demand proper training and are very effective for conditions such as musculoskeletal problems. They are sometimes used together alongside acupuncture treatment.

Gua Sha. Plum Blossom Needling

Both these therapies, which have been in use for centuries, create a rash on the skin. In fact the word "Sha" actually means a rash whereas "Gua" means to scrape. Treatment involves the scraping of the skin so a rash appears which stimulates the Qi energy. It is especially helpful for colds and flu symptoms, joint conditions as well as asthma, bronchitis, insomnia and post viral syndromes. Traditionally, it was used by the elderly as a form of preventive medicine, for health maintenance and to invigorate the system. It uses a blunt flat implement to produce the rash which is painless but which can remain on the skin for a few days before eventually fading.

Plum Blossom Needling, also called "Seven Star Hammer Therapy", uses a type of small hammer containing five or seven needle points which, when rapidly tapped on the surface of the skin, produces a rash similar to Gua Sha. The difference is that Plum Blossom Needling focuses on a local area or on a small number of acupuncture points rather than scraping over a larger area like Gua Sha. The needles don't penetrate the skin but produce a rash when tapped and has a similar effect as Gua Sha and is used for similar conditions. Traditionally it is used to treat children, the elderly and those patients who are apprehensive about having acupuncture treatment.

Quite often a Traditional Acupuncturist will incorporate cupping, some ear acupuncture, Gua Sha or massage, alongside their main emphasis of seeking the root cause of a patient's problems.

Emperors, The Forbidden City, Heaven, Earth and Humankind

The human being was considered of such importance that the ancient Chinese drew a parallel between its inner workings and those of their own kingdom, particularly their palaces. It was believed that balance, harmony and order within each leads to peace, health and prosperity in both. The vast palace known as the Forbidden City in Beijing, epitomises this extraordinary and unique correlation. In this chapter I have attempted to illustrate this with information gained from my visit there in November 1984 together with further research and observation. At its very centre was the Emperor, representing the Heart and under him were 11 Ministers, or court officials, corresponding to the other nine organs and two functions. Chinese writing, which uses pictures rather than words, portrays these organs in a rather wonderful way: they show a willing and obedient servant leaning towards the Emperor, eager to serve him and the empire and, by extension, us as human beings.

Provided these Ministers worked harmoniously together in carrying out his commands and the Emperor himself was stable and virtuous, the Empire flourished. However, if there was disharmony within the Empire, with an Emperor unfit to rule and who no longer had the support of his Ministers conflict and war would ensue. To take this analogy further, this disharmony would produce disease and illness within the empire of the human being.

In a more modern context, the workings of these 11 Ministers can be likened to a football team which has 11 players under the direction of their Manager. When a team is playing well the camaraderie is felt clearly by each player as they work together, often with a sort of intuition and perception borne of this team spirit and the game is a delight to watch. The Manager who, although not actively playing, is intrinsically involved in every aspect of the game and this invisible, but essential "team spirit" arises partly from his focus, inspiration and "presence". However, when there is conflict within the team, with a manager lacking in these qualities, this *esprit de corps* vanishes and usually results in the game being lost, or as in the earlier analogy, as illness arising within the human being.

Emperors

There have been Emperors in China since time immemorial and for its people he was the ruler of their world whose power covered "everything under heaven". The most ancient records refer to those who lived in the Shang dynasty (c. 1700–c.1100 BCE) as it was from this era that the first written records of the Chinese language originated; so it can be seen that they have been there as a powerful influence for nearly 4000 years. Before them there were others including five mythical Emperors, the most famous of these being the Yellow Emperor after whom the *Nei Jing* is named.

The most powerful and heartless of them all was probably Qin Shihuangdi who, in 221 BCE unified into one nation the 6 warring states that existed at that time and after whom China is named (Qin is pronounced Chin). It was he who extended the Great Wall and whose tomb is protected by the renowned Terra Cotta army. This army, made up of around 8,000 unique and varied warrior figures and positioned a mile to the east of the main tomb which it guards has yet to be opened. However, there are over 600 peripheral pits surrounding it that have been excavated. Some contain these warriors with others housing miniature palaces, vast numbers of exquisite porcelain objects and fabulous jewelry.

There are court acrobats to entertain him in the afterlife and elegant bronze carriages and horses all of which can only be an indication of the wonders that must lie within. An historian named Sima Qian later recorded that it contains a miniature working model of China with flowing rivers of mercury, representing the main rivers of China and above a replica of the constellations that could be seen at that time made of precious jewels. There are thought to be whale oil candles lit to last for eternity, and crossbows set to kill any tomb raiders who dared to force entry. It took seven hundred thousand men 38 years to build and at its completion hundreds of officials, concubines and labourers who knew its secrets were buried alive within it. But as fate would have it, Qin Shihuangdi himself died early at the age of 50 during an expedition, ironically, to find the elusive elixir of life; a dynasty that was intended to last 10,000 generations in reality only lasted 14 years.

It was during this time of great upheaval that Qin, in 213 BCE, ordered the mass burning of all books that were in circulation at that time and had buried alive many intellectuals who were critical of him in order to strengthen his own position as the legitimate ruler. However, those written about medicine, agriculture and divination were spared, the most important of these being the *Nei Jing*. It was from this time onwards that what we know as Chinese medicine, particularly acupuncture, moxibustion and herbal medicine became increasingly available throughout China. They would eventually be used over the following centuries to treat millions, perhaps billions of its people. These numbers may sound excessive but there have always been a lot of people living in China. This fact is illustrated by the world's earliest surviving large scale census there which gave the taxable population in 2 CE as 57,671,400.

Following Qin Shihuangdi's reign there have been a further 557 Emperors of China all with varying degrees of ability in ruling their vast empire and spanning a period of well over 2000 years. These Emperors were all expected to lead a life of complex ritual and ceremony as well as fulfilling their demanding administrative duties. These rites, of which there were around 150, determined his style of dress which had to correspond to the colour of each season, and how he received and entertained foreign envoys. They laid down the procedures to follow after bad harvests and illness and how he should conduct himself during the many ceremonies he had to carry out. These included marking the winter solstice, promulgating the calendar for the New Year, symbolically ploughing the first three furrows at the Altar of the Earth in Springtime and praying for good harvests at the Temple of Heaven. They even determined how he ate and how he regulated his sex life so that the right timing, predicted by the Court astrologers, would produce a son. No wonder some of them were unable to handle this weight of responsibility which placed such a great demand on their personal life and as a consequence lost their sanity. There was one Ming ruler who became so fed up and wearied by the incessant demands of running the Empire that he handed it all over to his officials and took up carpentry instead! Another withdrew into his Inner Court and refused to grant an audience or sign a document for 25 years. Others devoted their time to leisures and pleasures but there were many who were extraordinarily hard-working, talented, energetic and able who began their day at 4 am meeting with their senior Ministers and retired to bed at 8 pm.

Since the time of Confucius, (551–479 BCE), perhaps the most influential person in their history, it was believed that Heaven, Earth and human kind were all interconnected and that the Emperor, as "Son of Heaven", was deemed responsible for maintaining the delicate balance between these earthly and heavenly realms. Provided his behaviour was correct and virtuous then the Heavens would respond benevolently. As a result he would be granted the authority to govern through the "Mandate of Heaven" bestowed upon him by powers from a higher realm.

If, on the other hand, the Emperor did not fulfil his responsibilities correctly or became corrupt or tyrannical, Heaven would respond accordingly. This could take the form of earthquakes, floods, famine, fire , drought, or civil unrest. These would be construed as a sign that he had lost the "Mandate of Heaven" was no longer able to govern in accordance with Heaven's will, was inadequate for the task and thus could be removed from power. Some upright and courageous court officials even risked death by standing up to the Emperor to enforce this ancient Confucian right.

The Forbidden City

In 1420 CE, after 14 years of intense construction, employing a million labourers and a hundred thousand artisans the immense Imperial Palace, known today as The Forbidden City but also named the Purple City or the Great Within, was built in what was to be the new capital of China, Beijing. It was itself an inner city, surrounded by two even more vast ones and constructed on the same site where Kublai Khan had positioned his winter capital in 1267 CE. It was built to house the Ming Emperors and would become the seat of power for the whole of China and its Empire which would eventually influence much of Asia. China was by far the most populous and wealthiest nation in the world at that time and 24 Emperors would all rule from the Forbidden City, the last one abdicating in 1912. It was during the early part of this dynasty that the many aspects of Chinese medicine flourished and reached new heights of refinement. An example of this are the three acupuncture charts illustrated in this book which were drawn during this era.

This city, like those of previous ancient Chinese capitals, including the famous Xanandu immortalised by the poet Coleridge, was laid out following the strict laws of geomancy (known as Feng Shui). This is the science of placing manmade structures in harmony with the vital cosmic energy coursing through the earth, in order to create balance and harmony within it. Everything in the City's design had a symbolic meaning, from the number of gold bosses on the massive red gates, the colour of the roof tiles, to the position of its main hall which aligned with the Pole star, a celestial metaphor for the Emperor's role as central to the Empire. The most potent and auspicious of all these symbols is the Dragon. It is found throughout this city and was the prime embodiment of the heavenly energies working through the earth which, since the

Emperor's role was to mediate between the two, was also the embodiment of Imperial power and hence the Imperial emblem. The city is positioned on a north-south axis with the central meridian passing through the central portal of the Meridian Gate. It also passes through the centre of the Dragon Throne in the Hall of Supreme Harmony, the most eminent building in the whole of China. During important ceremonies the Emperor sat on the Dragon Throne which was placed upon a square dais, signifying the Earth, with a circular ceiling adorned with dragon and pearl symbols above representing the Heavens. Either side of the throne stood crane statues representing longevity and, wearing the ceremonial yellow silk dragon robe emblazoned with celestial emblems, dragons and the Five Elements, the Emperor was at the centre of the Empire. In this way he was symbolically uniting the worlds of Heaven, Earth and Man — the Heart of the whole universe.

Thus, with this auspicious design, the workings of the Imperial administration would enhance, reflect and be in harmony with the will of Heaven. The final consequence and ultimate aim was that, with a virtuous Emperor ruling under the "mandate of heaven", from a city laid out in a cosmically correct manner Heaven, Earth and its people would flourish in peace and harmony.

Heaven, Earth and Humankind

Hidden within the design of the Forbidden City the architect had placed another which is believed to correlate the structures and spaces of the city with those of the human body. Humankind was considered the most important of all beings in creation. Formed from the union of Heaven and Earth, whose highest representation was in the person of the Emperor it contained within it the highest manifestation of these two powers known in Chinese as *Shen* and in English as "the Spirits". The organs, too, were believed to contain a divine principle. This makes the design and its physiological representation even more extraordinary illustrating as it does the glory of the Empire, its ruler and the human being.

Set into the defensive walls of the outer city were placed nine gates representing the nine portals or orifices of the human body. This was also the number allocated solely to the Emperor. Further into the complex is the vast Tiananmen Square known in English as the Gate of Heavenly Peace from where Chairman Mao first proclaimed the founding of the People's Republic of China in 1949. Leading out of this square is the Meridian Gate, the main entrance into the inner city. Set into this gate are five entrances representing the Five Elements, three of which form the central portals signifying Heaven, Humankind and Earth.

After passing through these gates one enters another vast courtyard followed by a stream over which are five white marble bridges. These signify to some the five Confucian virtues and to others the five human senses which then lead into the core of the city or, in this case, the inner body itself.

Positioned at the very centre of it and set upon a three tiered marble terrace are three structures (the number 3, which is extensively used in this complex, represents the power of Heaven, Earth and Humankind). These three structures are represented within the ideogram of the Heart (see Diagram 7, below). This depicts the empty vessel of the Heart, the long line, above which are three shorter ones. These convey an understanding of the Heart's role as instrumental in the outward communication with both the Empire and the Human Body. The largest and most important of these three structures is the Hall of Supreme Harmony, signifying the Heart itself. It was from this Hall that the Emperor issued commands to his Ministers upon whose robes were sewn silk insignia indicating their status. They stood on flagstones in front of him, each marked in bronze according to their rank in the hierarchy for the

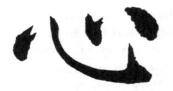

Diagram 7

daily running of the Empire. Each Minister present was required to kowtow or prostrate themselves three times and knock their foreheads on the flagstones nine times as a mark of respect for the Emperor before this dawn audience with him began.

The Ministers in their turn would pass on these Imperial edicts to their subordinates and so on down the line until eventually the most outlying communities of the Empire would be informed of and be regulated by the Emperor's commands. Thus cohesion and order be it of a city, village, family or individual would be maintained. The human analogy here is of the Heart rhythmically issuing life-giving sustenance via the Blood to the 11 Organs represented by those Ministers positioned on their flagstones and eventually to the farthest extremities of the Empire of the body. This applied both in a physical and spiritual sense because the Emperor was seen as the spiritual seat of power within the Empire. This fact is mirrored in Chinese Medicine by the role of the Heart which houses, protects and from it emanates the *Shen* or Spirit of a person whose quality is transported by the Blood throughout the body. It is this "shen" within the human body that differentiates us from all other beings in the animal kingdom and whose presence imparts glory and brilliance to each one of us.

Just as the Blood returns to the Heart to be revitalised, so the reports and petitions from the four corners of the Empire flowed back to the Emperor. They were read by him, marked with red ink and then acted upon; thus the Empire, as well as the human being, would flourish and be at peace — the ultimate aim of any virtuous ruler. The analogy here for us is the need to keep our own Hearts in a balanced and peaceful state so that the rest of us can thrive, which in this day and age, is no mean feat. However we can at least try and keep our consciousness clear and our spirits up so that we as individuals may flourish and live in peace — the ultimate aim of any virtuous medical system and its practitioner.

The tiered terrace which surrounds these three structures is named the Dragon Pavement. It represents the Pericardium, the protective tissue surrounding the Heart, known also as the

Heart Protector: an important function in Chinese Medicine which offers emotional as well as physical protection. Another Hall, known variously as the Hall of Union, the Hall of Vigorous Activity or the Hall of Vigorous Fertility which is positioned between the Palace of Heavenly Purity, (the residence of the Emperor,) and the Palace of Earthly Tranquillity (the residence of the Empress), represents an important acupuncture point. It lies between the two Kidneys and its name in Classical Acupuncture is the *Gate of Life*. One of the functions of this point is to help in treating cases of infertility. Other buildings with names such as the Hall of Central Harmony, the Pavilion of Pleasant Sounds, Nurturing the Heart Hall and the Hall of Mental Cultivation together with others that represent the intestines and viscera further illustrate the physiological analogy woven into this design.

Thus we can see the correlation between the macrocosmic heavenly city, itself representing the universe, and the microcosmic earthly human being. Both correspond to and function symbiotically together via the spiritual pivot of the Heart/Emperor.

This observation of the human being, the discovery and unravelling of the meridian system within it and the understanding of the complex action of the acupuncture points, which you will read about later in the book, is a magnificent achievement. It can be said to compare in magnitude to the sequencing of the human genome in today's world.

The following chapter on each of the Elements describes how they and their associated organs and functions can become imbalanced. It shows how you can recognise these signs and, with the aid of the questionnaire that relates to each Element together with the accompanying recommendations, how they can then be regulated. It will also give you a flavour of each of them, and, bearing in mind that they are all encompassed within us, you will see that you have your own personal connection with them.

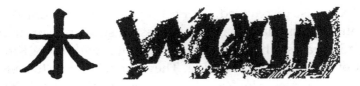

The Wood Element

Acupuncture point names associated with this Element include: *Upright Living, Sun and Moon, Bright and Clear, Great Esteem, Happy Calm, Gate of Hope, Hasty Pulse, Insect Ditch.*

Wood governs the function of the Liver and Gallbladder.

The Liver does many things but its primary tasks are to break down fatty foods and remove toxins from the bloodstream.

The ancient Oriental medical tradition, though, gives the Liver a much wider sphere of influence which here in the West, we are only just beginning to understand. An Oriental physician will gauge the health of your Liver by looking out for certain classic signs. These include frontal headaches, pain behind the eyes, muscular spasms, high blood pressure, itchiness in sensitive areas, blurred vision, painful periods or pains just below the rib cage. Excessive anger, a shouting voice, irritability or a greenish hue on the face may also point to a Liver that's in need of attention. (A Western doctor, reading this list, would also recognize some — though not all — of these symptoms as being Liver related.)

If you do tend to suffer from any of the above, the suggestions outlined below could prove especially useful to you.

The Chinese discovered, over centuries of observation, that the Liver and its associated energy are responsible for our ability to plan and organise things, seeing its function within the Kingdom as that of a Minister of Planning. They likened it also to a General in the armed forces who 'excelled at strategic planning'. This militaristic association is also reflected in the expression "Gung Ho" which is Chinese for "Fire in the Liver". The Liver helps us to 'see in our mind's eye' the way forward in our lives. It is also the source of our ability to put these plans into action and when we do so, we begin to grow with confidence. If our Liver energy remains healthy, we naturally organize our life better so that it flows more smoothly and our goals are more likely to be achieved.

If this growth is thwarted, however, we may experience irritability, anger (which is the main emotion associated with the Wood Element), a feeling of hopeless despair or a lack of direction in our lives. Various factors can contribute to the development of a Wood imbalance, but often it will occur when we let something else take control of our lives. This can be a person, a situation or a habitual indulgence in some kind of drug.

On a more physical level, a Wood imbalance can result in headaches or migraine, eye disorders and menstrual problems as well as a feeling of being 'snarled up within', when life is just not going our way. Furthermore, our planning and judgemental abilities become affected and we often make mistakes regarding our careers, relationships or general direction in life.

The other organ associated with the Wood Element is the Gallbladder.

On a strictly Western medical level the Gallbladder stores bile which aids in the digestion of foods, especially fats. But again Chinese Medicine sees its influence as being much greater than this. Since ancient times it has been seen as the Minister responsible for co-ordination, judgement and decision-making. If the Gallbladder energy is imbalanced we can experience confusion, indecision, lack of clarity or poor judgement. Other more physical symptoms can be digestive disorders, one-sided headaches, arthritis, particularly of the hips and knees, eye problems and a tendency to become accident-prone due to a lack of co-ordination. If these imbalances carried on for many years then it's conceivable they could lead to more serious conditions associated with the Liver and Gallbladder later on in life. However, well before these conditions arise we can take steps to avoid them. The highest form of medicine is preventive medicine which was a fact noted many centuries ago in a famous Chinese quote which said: 'going to a doctor when you're ill is like a thirsty person digging a well'. In other words it's too late and that "an ounce of prevention is worth a ton of cure".

Balancing your Wood Element

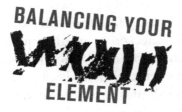

i) Try and cut down on fatty foods such as cheese, fish and chips and cream.

ii) Try to moderate your alcohol intake because the Liver has to detoxify it.

iii) Avoid sour foods like vinegar.

iv) If you are taking presciption drugs, see if your doctor can reduce your dosage. This is particularly relevant if you are on repeat prescriptions, where a re-assessment hasn't been made for a number of months. Any reduction, **safely made**, and monitored by your physician would be of benefit.

v) Ensure you have a regular intake of zinc, calcium and vitamin B2, especially if your nails are of poor quality and have white patches on them. (Oysters contain the highest amount of zinc followed by wheatgerm, bran and sesame seeds.)

vi) In windy, cold weather always make sure the back of your neck is covered by a warm scarf as this helps protect your

Gallbladder energy from wind or cold attack which can enter into the system through a point on the neck called *Wind Gate*.

vii) If your anger and irritability is causing you concern, try lying down quietly with your hands over your lower ribcage. Use a relaxation tape and concentrate on that region. Visualize calm and peaceful feelings entering your body there. Alternatively, you can safely release pent-up anger by having a large pillow or cushion at hand and giving it a good, thorough pummelling. Traditional Acupuncture can also help effectively with excessive anger. It's not that anger is wrong; it's the degree of it, what we do with it and what we can learn from it that are the issues.

viii) Try hypnotherapy, Tai Qi, yoga or meditation to help you feel more relaxed and balanced.

ix) For mild indecision take the Bach Flower Remedy Scleranthus. For chronic indecision consult a qualified acupuncturist.

x) For migraine and headaches, press gently but firmly on the area of your temple towards the eye bones. Do this for just one or two minutes at a time, always applying the pressure to both sides. . . while keeping your eyes closed.

xi) Gardening or growing indoor plants could be a good, supportive way to enhance your Wood energy.

xii) Try playing Monopoly or chess (good for decision making and planning), but don't get angry if you lose!

xiii) During the winter months, conserve your energy as best you can. Go to bed earlier and get up later. This in turn will help your energy during the spring, which is the season associated with Wood.

xiv) For muscular, ligament or tendon problems which are commonly associated with the Wood Element, deep remedial massage is recommended.

xv) Your eyes have a close connection to the Wood Element, particularly the Liver. Get a regular check-up at the optician's at least once a year. Alternatively, you might consider the Bates method to help eye weaknesses.

xvi) Certain foods support and strengthen your Wood:

- Cereals such as wheat, oats, barley and rye;
- Pulses, especially green lentils, mung beans and black eyed beans;
- Vegetables, such as globe artichokes, green peppers, broccoli, leeks, raw carrot, lettuce, parsley, runner beans and peas ;
- Also fruits, including apples, avocadoes, citrus fruits, pineapples and plums.
- Herbs that are 'good for Wood' include marjoram, cumin, caraway, bay leaf, tarragon, cloves. And if you need a source of protein, try Brazil or cashew nuts or free range poultry.

xvii) Try to avoid foods and drinks with a lot of chemicals in them. (The Liver has to de-toxify these.)

xviii) Eat organically grown foods as much as possible for this same reason. Current research suggests that chemicals in our food could alter a person's DNA, or even the more complex histone coding, which in turn affects our genetic structure and perhaps an individual's susceptibility to disease.

xix) Some Feng Shui practitioners specialise in the Five Element tradition. It may be worth finding such an expert and inviting them to help show you how to re-arrange your home so that it becomes more supportive of your Wood Element.

xx) If your need becomes more acute, you might consult a qualified healer in therapies such as Acupuncture, Reflexology, Shiatsu or Chinese Herbal Medicine.

xxi) Another cause of a Wood imbalance can arise from our experiences of anger or repressed anger. During childhood our slates are pretty clean, so if, for instance, we experienced a lot of anger or bullying at this time this could eventually disturb our Wood Element, particularly the Liver. These experiences could, later on, result in ourselves becoming full of anger, or conversely repressing it within, both of which would have an adverse affect on this Element. However, if you do have a history of inappropriate anger or irritability, particularly towards another person, then forgiveness can work wonders. It's easier said than done, but with some good counselling, Traditional Acupuncture or guided imagery, this problem could be helped a lot.

xxii) Any type of racquet sport would be a good hobby to get into as they help to release physical and mental tension.

xxiii) You might consider trying Traditional Chinese healing music incorporating the Cheuh tone. Therapeutically it is recommended for many symptoms associated with imbalances in the Wood Element including digestive problems, excessive anger, low libido, lack of motivation, impotence and irritability. More information on this is given in the chapter on Preventive Medicine.

An Example of a Wood CF

Hannah, aged 46, a secondary school teacher, had come primarily with one-sided migraines which produced severe pain behind her left eye and had troubled her on a regular basis since her teens. Her secondary problems were disturbed sleep, irrritability (particularly around period time), difficulties forming plans or solutions for the future and intermittent digestive pains all of which made her tense and on edge.

During the consultation it transpired that her father had also suffered from migraines and that, like Hannah, had hated the wind which would make them worse. Her childhood had been generally unhappy as a result of her father needing to continually control her and for the fact that he would often be angry but in a repressed sort of manner. Hannah would also regularly crave cheese and other fatty foods which she thought might be the cause of her indigestion and which could, at times, trigger a migraine. Her voice was lacking in strength and around her eyes, towards the outer edge, there was a slighly greenish hue. Her emotions were dominated by continual feelings of anger and irritability which she mostly suppressed.

The diagnosis was that Hannah's main area of weakness lay in her Wood Element, specifically her Gallbladder energy, rather than her Liver.

Although it is sometimes hard to differentiate between the two it was the one-sidedness of the migraine that pointed towards the Gallbladder rather than the Liver, both of which make up the Wood Element. This was also an example of an hereditary condition passed on from her father and exacerbated by his need to continually control her all of which had contributed to this disturbance in her Gallbladder energy.

Hannah was advised to reduce her intake of fatty foods, especially cheese and after seven or eight treatments supporting her Wood Element, particularly the Gallbladder, she found that her one-sided migraines were much less severe and much less frequent. She also found that her decision-making and future planning abilities improved and after some weeks realised her sleep was better too. This latter improvement was more to do with the fact that her practitioner was also treating her Liver energy, whose height of functioning is between 1 am and 3 am. She was also less irritable around the period time, again as a result of work on the Liver energy and later on she felt more able to begin the process of reconciliation with her father. Hannah continued coming for maintenance treatment about five times a year at the change of the seasons to prevent her symptoms returning and also to keep her functioning at her optimum best.

WOOD ELEMENT QUESTIONNAIRE

In each section, you will find 15 questions that relate to different aspects of each of the Elements. Just read each one and give your immediate, honest answer. Don't stop and think for too long. Your first impulsive reaction to the questions is almost certainly the most useful one. Tick the box beside your answer — or keep a tally of the number of A's, B's, and C's. At the end, we'll be able to see what they reveal about your relationship to each Element. Even if some questions seem too specific just go with the one most applicable to you.

1) How do you like the colour green?

    A. It's always been my clear favourite.
    B. It's OK.
    C. Don't like it at all. I would never wear it or paint my walls with it.

Green is a springtime colour, symbolic of lively, dynamic growth. The Wood Element is strongly linked to green.

2) How do you like sour tastes (such as pickled onions?)

    A. I eat them nearly every day.
    B. Only occasionally.
    C. I won't touch them, they make me feel ill.

Some people like vinegar so much, they are tempted to drink it! If your Wood Energy is out of balance, you will probably have a strong reaction one way or another, to sour tastes.

3) How are you when it comes to making decisions?

    A. I always find it easy.
    B. I usually find it easy.
    C. I'm not quite sure whether I'm decisive or not. Probably, I'm not.

Since ancient times, the ability to make decisions has been recognised as being governed by the Gallbladder.

4) How is your ability to plan for future events and activities?

    A. Very good. My diary is full of firm, long term commitments.
    B. Fairly good — but I am happy to be flexible.
    C. Not so great. I really do try to make plans but somehow, I just can't.

The ability to plan and organise is traditionally associated with the Liver.

5) Would you call yourself a good organiser?

    A. Most definitely. I simply can't abide living with messy arrangements as I always need to be in control of the situation.

    B. Maybe. I can normally manage to get things together.

    C. Not at all. I seem to be constantly disorganised.

The Liver is the body's 'military general'. To be a successful administrator you need to have your 'Liver energy' in good order.

6) How are your fingernails at the moment?

    A. Hard as diamonds.

    B. Generally strong and flexible.

    C. Brittle with a tendency to break easily and/or develop white spots.

Our nails sit at the very extremities of our body. They grow strongly and slowly, rather like the branches of a tree. This may be why the ancients saw them as linked, so strongly, to the Wood Element).

7) How is your self-esteem?

    A. My self-esteem is just fine thanks. How is yours?

    B. Reasonably good — but we're none of us perfect.

    C. Not so good — I'm very self-critical and don't have much confidence in myself at all.

A tree has no doubt about what it is — and why it exists. It follows an organic impulse to grow in a very particular, pre-defined way. People with a good 'Wood balance' have a similar tendency to feel naturally self-confident.

8) When you feel you need a little extra luck . . . or you make a statement that you hope will always remain true, do you 'touch wood'?

    A. Every time. I really don't want things to go wrong for me.

    B. Maybe once in a while, but if I can't find anything wooden to touch I'm not too bothered.

C. I would never 'touch wood'. That's just silly and superstitious.

9) When you're out of doors on a windy day, how do you feel?

A. Delighted. I love a nice bracing breeze. It makes me feel invigorated.

B. Fine unless there's a really bitter, icy gale blowing.

C. Irritated, agitated. Strong winds can even give me a headache.

NB: If you picked C, here's a supplementary question. Have you particularly noticed that this is worse when there's an East wind blowing? If so, count your answer TWICE.

10) Is there a special time of day or night when you 'come alive' and feel especially creative?

A. Yes. It's often quite late. Between 11 pm and 1 am. Sometimes I can be up till 3 am cooking up ideas or even cleaning the home.

B. Not really, unless I've had a lot of cheese or alcohol.

C. I don't like to stay up late at night — I'm always asleep by 11 pm at the latest.

11) 'The world's favourite season is the spring. All things seem possible in May.' (Edwin Thomas.) Do you agree?

A. Very much so. Spring is my favourite season. I can't wait for it to arrive.

B. Not especially. Spring is a lovely season — but then there's magic at every time of year.

C. Not at all. I can never understand why people get so excited about this season.

Spring is the season associated with Wood.

12) Do you easily cry?

A. I can burst into tears at the drop of a hat. I often cry when I'm angry too — probably out of sheer frustration.

B. Only occasionally.

C. I hardly ever let myself cry.

Wood influences our level of emotional self-control. If imbalanced it can make us more prone to tears.

13) Do you often suffer from itchy skin?

   A. No.

   B. Not unless I've been bitten by something.

   C. Yes. Indeed, the very suggestion is enough to make me feel as though insects are crawling over me.

NB: Various medications can cause a skin reaction. Alcohol can also change your skin's sensitivity. Choose B. not C. if you suspect that either of these factors are giving you irritated skin.

14) How do you like cheese?

   A. I'm very partial to it; especially strong, creamy cheeses or the blue veined types.

   B. On a pizza or with pickle in a sandwich it can be quite nice sometimes.

   C. I really don't like it. It can give me indigestion or a headache; particularly the one-sided variety.

NB: Cheese, along with other fatty foods, is an interesting indicator of your 'Wood balance'. If the Wood Element within you is out of balance, you will either strongly crave — or react badly to — cheese in your diet.

15) Which of the following statements can you most easily relate to?

   A. I always like to know exactly what's what — and I like things to happen my way. If they don't I get angry or upset.

   B. I don't especially feel that I need to be in control all the time.

   C. I like to 'go with the flow'. I'd rather just adapt to what's happening. I don't want to be responsible for taking charge of anything or anyone.

Now add up your scores.

   No. of A. answers.

   No. of B. answers.

   No. of C. answers.

Conclusions

IF YOU HAVE MAINLY B's: Your Wood Element is pretty balanced. You're a clear thinker, intelligently decisive with good planning and organisational abilities. You have healthy eyes, good co-ordination and a comfortable level of emotional stability. You're good at expressing your anger in an appropriate way when it's justified — and at knowing how to keep your temper in check when it makes more sense to do so. You are reliable, hard working, and when you say you're going to do something, you do it. Because you are so well organised, you rarely find yourself feeling flummoxed or taken by surprise. You can cope with pressure, you like excitement and adventure — and you're very happy to take brave steps when you need to. Though you have a competitive edge to your personality, you're not insecure. If you encounter someone with a special talent or skill, you are far more likely to show supportive appreciation than to experience secret jealousy. Your friends, though, sometimes think that you can be a little too sure of yourself. Life for you is a process of discovery. You like to learn, you like to explore and you are always open to new ideas.

This does not mean, though, that your overall Oriental Element balance is in perfect shape. Over the remainder of this book there will be four more crucial checks to perform. Almost certainly, if you complete the other questionnaires, you'll find at least one Element which is a little out of kilter. When you do, you'll be able to read a list of practical suggestions to help bring harmony back into that important area of your life.

IF YOU HAVE MORE THAN EIGHT A's: You have a tendency to be a little accident prone. Things 'just happen' to you and you're never quite sure why. Nor are you quite sure how to react. You can be calm one moment yet furious the next and the emotion you display will often come as much as a surprise to you as it does to the person on the receiving end of it. In some ways though, you quite like being spontaneous. Life is exciting when it's surprising — and that's much the same reason why you rather enjoy doing things in a hurry or taking unnecessary risks. You thrive on pressure, you're always in a hurry, there are never enough hours in the day and you're probably a very successful person. This success though, may well come about 'in spite of' rather than because of your impatience. If you can learn to balance out your Wood energy, by following the steps below, you will discover that you can accomplish far, far more. Please read the advice carefully and slowly — but I know that you never really do anything carefully and slowly. Nonetheless, please try to pay as much attention as you currently can!

IF YOU HAVE MORE THAN EIGHT C's: You are a very special person — perhaps far more special than you give yourself credit for being. For some reason, you tend to work against your own best interests, by criticising yourself too heavily or allowing yourself to feel as if you are just a helpless victim of circumstance. And yet, you can be very powerful and strong when you need to be. The trouble is you get excited — or fired up with energy — only to find that you can't quite maintain your mood for as long as you need to. Nothing ever stays the same in your life for too long and you're full of hopes and ideas that never really come to much. It's all a great shame because you undoubtedly have a tremendous potential to achieve great things. If you can only re-adjust your level of Wood energy, you will be able to lead a much calmer, more controlled, more satisfying existence. And you can. All you have to do is overcome that little voice of doubt which, even now, as you read this, is saying 'this system will not work for me'. It will. So please, do go on to read the section below.

IF YOU HAVE MORE THAN EIGHT A's OR MORE THAN EIGHT C's: There is clearly some degree of imbalance in your Wood Element. It's quite normal to have at least one Element that's in need of some attention but it is also desirable to do something about it. Please consult the self-help section.

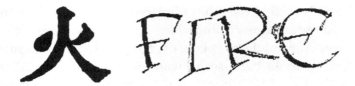

火 FIRE

The Fire Element

Acupuncture point names associated with this Element include: *Spirit Gate, Nourishing the Old, Heavenly Ancestor, The Intermediary, Palace of Weariness, Relax and Joy, Listening Palace, Ear Gate.*

Contained within this Element are two organs — the Heart and Small Intestine — and two functions — the Three Heater and the Heart Protector (known also as the Pericardium). Whereas Wood is the Element of dynamic growth, Fire is concerned with passion, joy, maturity and sexuality. In this section we will be looking at ourselves from another angle and gaining more insight into this different aspect of our make-up .

First of all, let's look at the Heart. As was mentioned before, the ancient Chinese saw the human being as a Kingdom with an Emperor who had eleven Ministers under him, each of whom had specific functions and responsibilities within it. They likened the Heart to their Emperor because he presided over their Kingdom and whose authority extended to all corners of the land just as its action moves blood to the smallest capillaries of the extremities. Everything was fine if the Emperor was in good health and, as a result, all the Ministers under him would work well together as a team. However, if the Emperor wasn't in good health, that in turn would be conveyed to the other Ministers, and so on down the line until the Kingdom wasn't flourishing so well any more.

The Emperor should be fit in body, mind and spirit — particularly in the last attribute because he was seen as the spiritual seat of power in the Kingdom and acted as the intermediary between the Heavens and the people on the Earth. The 'radiance of the spirit emanate from it' refers to the microcosmic connection with our own inbuilt higher consciousness. We know what happens when an Emperor loses his sense of balance (the Chinese interpretation of this state was that he had 'lost the mandate of Heaven'): the Kingdom degenerates into chaos meaning, in this case, ill health and disease.

Now the Emperor was considered so important that he had a Protector or a sort of Praetorian Guard around him. This is called the Heart Protector, or to use another name for it: the Pericardium meridian. We will talk more about this fascinating function later on. After that comes the Small Intestine, which separates and transforms into energy the food and drink we take into our bodies. Finally comes the fourth part of the Fire Element — the Three Heater whose function is responsible for maintaining the correct temperature within us both physically and emotionally. It also helps distribute the Qi energy evenly throughout the body which in turn keeps our immune system in good shape. Being "in charge of the waterways" of the body, the regulation of its fluids stem from this complex meridian also.

Please complete the 15-part questionnaire now on page 62.

The Four Parts of Fire

We talked about the Heart earlier on, but what happens when this important function gets out of balance? We can experience being easily shocked, on edge and often confused as well as getting frequent panic attacks or feeling anxious at the slightest thing. A lot of stress placed upon the system, an excessive work load with no time to relax combined with bad eating and drinking habits, can bring this about. Taking steps now to regulate and moderate our lifestyle will help to avoid more serious Heart problems in the future.

The Small Intestine, which is closely connected to the Heart (their structural material is very similar) is a highly intelligent part of our anatomy. Its ministerial functions are that of 'separating the pure from the impure' and 'making things thrive' within the Kingdom. Everything that we eat or drink gets sorted out here as it throws out stuff that is no good to us, and retains the good, which it sends to the Spleen who then transforms it into pure energy. And it's all done automatically! So if this organ is working well we get what we need and don't get what we don't need. However, if it's not working harmoniously, it doesn't throw out all the bad stuff and can throw out some of the good stuff too which can result in skin eruptions, noises in the ear, digestive problems, nutrient deficiencies and arthritis. On the mental/emotional levels this imbalance can cause mental confusion or a 'woolly head' when it can even feel like a physical effort to think straight or to sort things out in our mind. In this day and age the Small Intestine comes under increasing pressure with all the sorting out we have to do. This arises particularly from the most common daily activities of shopping, processing information from the computer and television screens, reading newspapers, and conversing on our mobile phones. It also affects our ability to discriminate, and for this reason plays a major role in our moral 'uprightness'.

The third part of the Fire Element is the function mentioned before — the Heart Protector. One of its ministerial functions is to 'infuse the Kingdom with elation and joy'. Just as we have a physical protection for the Heart called the pericardium, so we have an emotional protection too. This other function protects the Heart from the 'slings and arrows' that are constantly levelled at us, particularly on the emotional/relationship side of our lives. In fact, the term 'a broken Heart' refers not to the Heart itself but to this protector of it. This is what gets affected when we experience lack of love or rejection in our lives, especially as a child, or a break-down in our close relationships.

Our sexuality, as we know, is closely linked to intimacy, warmth and love, and the ability to express these things is also partly governed by this function. Through unhappy experiences to do with affairs of the Heart, sexual repression or abuse we can become over-vulnerable and withdrawn, which can result in our sexuality becoming distorted. It can then turn from being a source of pleasure and fulfillment to a feeling of being snarled up, furtive or dirty. However, when this function is well balanced we feel much more at ease, particularly with the social and sexual side of our make-up, and have no need to put up barriers in order to protect ourselves.

The last part of the Fire Element is the other function and is called the Three Heater or Triple Burner. It works like a bodily thermostat, maintaining our whole system at an even temperature which has to be kept very exact or we start to feel a bit 'off'. The Three Heater is the Minister in charge of the central heating system of the body and in addition helps to regulate and distribute the bodily fluids throughout it. When this function is out of balance, we can experience fluctuations in temperature when one part of us is warm and another cold such as hot flushes or cold hands and feet.

A balanced Three Heater keeps us emotionally balanced too but when it goes off-kilter we can experience blowing hot and cold emotionally. One moment we're the life and soul of the party, full of the joys of spring, and the next we're feeling dejected and lacking in joy. Furthermore this extraordinary meridian has a great influence on how we interact and communicate with people.

Self-Help Suggestions to Support and Strengthen your Fire Element

BALANCING YOUR

FIRE

ELEMENT

i) Whisky, Brandy and spirits in general would not be good for your system as they create a lot of heat in the body. Try and cut them out for a few weeks and you'll feel the benefit. The same applies to sugar and sugary foods and drinks.

ii) Try to moderate your intake of hot, spicy foods like curries, chillies, black pepper, butter, coffee and red meats, particularly if you are a person who gets a lot of heat in your body.

iii) Foods that would support your Fire are rice, corn, milk, carrots, and onions.

iv) Try not to have very hot baths or saunas, because this excessive heat would not be so good for your Fire, particularly if you scored mostly A's in the questionnaire.

v) Tai Chi, Qi Gong and Yoga would be good things to get involved in, because they calm and balance the system.

vi) If you don't get to laugh much, try to rekindle that side of your life by, for instance, getting in some hilarious movies or reading something humorous.

vii) If you're on your own and have the time, think about keeping a pet — they can bring warmth, calmness, affection and love and don't usually answer back!

viii) Try and keep your food and drink as free as possible from chemicals and toxins — changing to organic foods would be a good start. This puts less strain on your Small Intestine, which is concerned with separating the pure from the impure.

ix) Try treating yourself to at least one fun thing a week, like going to a movie, taking dancing lessons or buying that one small thing you've been putting off for no known reason!

x) If you have had problems with relationships in the past or are just plain shy and vulnerable, then good counselling, psychotherapy or Traditional Acupuncture could be helpful and supportive to you.

xi) Relaxed, focused hobbies like watercolour painting or cross-stitching could also be good for you.

xii) For men, try to regulate your sex life — too much can have a negative effect on the system. For centuries, the Chinese have laid down a general guideline for the **maximum** number of ejaculations at a certain age that would be considered healthy: at age 20 twice a day; at 30 once a day; at 40 once every three days; at 50 every five days; at 60 every ten days and at 70, every 30 days. If you're not in good health, or are tired, then double the time. (e.g. at age 50, once every ten days etc.). But remember, these are simply guidelines written nearly 1500 years ago! The reason for this is that too frequent sexual activity can deplete what is known as our 'Jing', or Essence which is draining on the system and can eventually damage our health. A woman's *Jing*, incidentally, is partly lost in pregnancy and childbirth.

xiii) Try and cut down on stimulants such as coffee and strong Indian tea and replace them with herbal teas, rooibosch tea or Barleycup.

xiv) Try and cut down on activities that cause you to feel over-excited or hyper.

xv) A beneficial thing for you to do would be to sit around an open fire (preferably burning wood) either indoors or out as it would have a nourishing effect on your inner Fire.

xvi) Symptoms associated with the Three Heater, such as temperature irregularities, difficulty in interacting with people, or emotional instability, can often be helped by Traditional Acupuncture.

xvii) The musical tone which is most influential in harmonising the Fire Element is the Chiah tone and you might try out this form of music and see how it affects you.

Much of Chinese healing music is based on the Law of the Five Elements and has been composed in order to regulate the circulation of Qi in the human being. It is referred to in the *Nei Jing* and can help improve the function of the internal organs (including the Heart Protector and Three Heater), strengthen psychological conditions and balance the emotions; further information is given in the Chapter on Preventive Medicine.

An Example of a Fire CF

Jonathan, aged 42 and unmarried, had suffered from severe acne since his late teens. He admitted that he was rather sceptical about acupuncture but had been recommended by a friend and was prepared to give it a go. He was at least open to it — a fact which is helpful for any practitioner, as it allows rapport, an essential ingredient in the therapeutic relationship, to flow between patient and practitioner. He had been working in hot kitchens at the time and was also constantly being made fun of by his co-workers which he found difficult to deal with. His strict all-male school environment and strong religious upbringing had furthermore resulted in him being unable to deal with relationships with the opposite sex.

His struggle here was that he couldn't reconcile his somewhat Victorian upbringing, which set its own standards as to how he should treat women, with the very different expectations of them in the modern world. On top of this lay his poor diet, especially being drawn to foods containing a lot of sugar, specifically liquorice. His facial colour was of a reddish hue and his voice was generally of a jovial nature; his body odour was that of newly ironed clothes, known to practitioners as a "scorched" odour, which relates to the Fire Element and which became more noticeable when he perspired.

His imbalance was in the Fire Element and it was the Small Intestine within it that had been weakened and was the one area most in need of treatment. On account of his mental and emotional stress over a considerable period of time his system had produced a negative form of energy known as "aggressive energy". The first treatment carried out by the practitioner was to remove this from his system. Further treatment was focussed on the Fire Element particularly the Small Intestine meridian. Jonathan was also advised by his practitioner to cut out all sweet things as they were producing heat within his system which, together with his job as a chef working in hot conditions, were exacerbating his condition.

In addition he took the advice of having a number of counselling sessions to help specifically with his relationship issues with women.

Some weeks later his skin condition improved to a degree where he was less troubled and stressed by it although it took another two months to improve further. He found that he was much brighter and more focussed within himself and was able to have more clarity regarding the direction in his life he wished to take. Additional treatment was on his Heart Protector meridian. This has an important role to play in relationship issues, which together with the counselling sessions he was receiving, helped him to be more at ease in his interactions with women.

He returns around five times a year for a seasonal check up and for the practitioner to keep a close eye on his Small Intestine energy. To date, his skin condition and more positive outlook on life continue to hold steady.

THE FIRE ELEMENT QUESTIONNAIRE

Below you will find 15 questions. Just read each one and give your immediate, honest answer as you did in the Wood section. At the end we will see what your responses reveal about your relationship with the Fire Element.

1) **How do you like the colour red?**

    A. My favourite colour. I love to wear it and have it in the house a lot.
    B. I quite like it.
    C. I never wear it — it's my least favourite colour.

Red is the colour of passion and the summertime. The Fire Element is strongly linked to red.

2) **How do you enjoy social events like parties?**

   A. I'm told I'm the life and soul of any party or celebration — but I often feel down afterwards.
   B. I quite like parties.
   C. I hate going to them — I'm very shy and always find it difficult to break the ice with strangers.

3) **How do you feel your bodily thermostat is?**

   A. I can overheat easily when other people seem to be much less hot. I also find I'm emotionally volatile too — one moment I'm up the next I'm down.
   B. I seem to adjust to a change in temperature quite well.
   C. I'm always cold and sometimes get chilblains in Winter.

4) **Do you like sorting drawers out?**

   A. I'm always doing it and really enjoy it.
   B. I do it sometimes.
   C. I never do it — I'm always in a muddle and can never get round to it. I don't know what to throw out or what to keep.

This ability can reflect the state of the functioning of the Small Intestine which discriminates between what is needed and what is not.

5) **Do you like spicy foods?**

   A. Love them — I have them quite a few times a week.
   B. I have them every now and then.
   C. Never have them — I feel hot and get tummy troubles after eating them.

6) **When you go shopping do you find you can't think straight after a short while?**

   A. No — I'm always clear-headed even after a day's shopping.
   B. I go that way occasionally.
   C. Very much so.

This can indicate the state of the functioning of the Small Intestine energy.

7) **Do you find it difficult to sort things out in your head?**

   A. I'm always very clear in my head even after a hard day's work.
   B. Only very rarely.
   C. Yes — very often I feel 'addled' in my head.

8) **How do you react to heat or hot weather in general?**

   A. I'm happiest in the hot summer — I just love it.
   B. I'm usually OK with it.
   C. Heat makes me feel a bit ill. I'm much better in the cool shade.

One of the Three Heater's function is to help the body adjust to temperature differences.

9) **How do you get on with other people?**

   A. I'm very easy going and get on well with most people I meet.
   B. I'm generally pretty OK in this area.
   C. I always find it very hard to open up to another person — let alone a group of people.

10) **Have you ever experienced a broken Heart and never feel to have got over it?**

   A. Yes.

   B. Yes but I got over it with the passage of time.

   C. I never let myself get too close to another person so I don't experience those feelings. I'm just too vulnerable.

11) **Do you get over-excited about things?**

   A. Yes — and I feel it's a bit over the top at times.

   B. I can get excited about things but it rarely feels excessive.

   C. I never get excited about anything — why should I? There's not much joy in this world is there?

12) **Do you like lying down?**

   A. I never do. I'm too bound up in rushing around I never have time.

   B. Occasionally.

   C. I do it whenever I can.

Fire people are often rushing around and will jump at the chance to lie down and rest.

13) **How often do you have a good laugh?**

   A. I need to get a laugh all the time — sometimes I feel a bit addicted to the feeling.

   B. I like a good laugh every now and then.

   C. I never have a laugh — what's there to laugh about — have you read the newspapers recently?

14) **If someone drops something behind your back do you jump out of your skin with fright?**

   A. Never — I'm always steady whatever happens.
   B. Very occasionally.
   C. Yes.

15) **Do you perspire easily?**

   A. I perspire a lot — even with the slightest exertion.
   B. It feels normal.
   C. I rarely perspire — even when I do some exercise.

Now add up your scores.
   No. of A. answers.
   No. of B. answers.
   No. of C. answers.

Conclusions

IF YOU HAVE MAINLY B's: Your Fire looks pretty balanced. You are good at communication without being too verbose, lively without being too excitable or, conversely, lacking in joy. You relish the excitement of social occasions and enjoy the empathy that can be created amongst people. Your discriminatory powers work well and, for the most part, your view of life is one of optimism.

IF YOU HAVE MAINLY A's: You are likely to be a very sensitive person who tends to wear their 'Heart on their sleeve'. Being so open, you can be vulnerable to other people's feelings, good or bad, and consequently suffer from the pain that this can bring. You would be helped by working on your emotional boundaries so that you get to know when to protect yourself and when to open up safely with others. Consult the list of suggestions to help give support to the Fire Element as this can only benefit the whole system.

IF YOU HAVE MAINLY C's: The indications are that this side of you is a little under par. You often find it difficult to sort things out in your life, whether it be at home in your relationships, or just life in general. You might need to work on being a little more open with people, as part of you might have shut down — perhaps because of previous hurtful experiences. With proper help, this can be done safely and allow you to interact more easily in the world.

Common physical symptoms of a Fire imbalance can be over-heating or poor circulation, tightness in the chest area or disturbed sleep. There can also be sexual problems like premature ejaculation or difficulties in maintaining an erection etc. or a coldness when it comes to anything of a sexual nature. Speech disorders and fluctuations in blood pressure can also be symptoms of an imbalance in this Element. Please follow the list of suggestions to help redress these imbalances. But remember, laughter is still one of the best medicines.

More on the Function of the Fire Ministers

The Heart governs all aspects of our blood, including its ability to propel it to the farthest extremities of our bodies via our arteries and the smallest of the capillaries. This gives rise to the analogy, mentioned earlier, of the Emperor having influence throughout the land. Being physically at the centre of the Kingdom he is aided in this task by the actions of his personal envoy, the Heart Protector/ the Pericardium official, whose job it is to manifest the radiance of the Heart/Emperor to the people. The organ associated to the Emperor, other than the Heart, is the tongue which can be seen as an organ of command and, interestingly, an imbalance in its function usually shows as a redness on the tip of the tongue.

The Small Intestine's responsibility is to sort everything out that we ingest. Within it lie huge numbers of villi which are little columns of hair-like structures that extend the surface area of this organ to a mind boggling 30 sq. yards — roughly the size of a garage. It is here that the processed food and liquid from the Stomach, passing through this forest of villi, gets sorted out. The pure substances are then passed on to the Spleen who transforms them into energy and then transports it around the body. The impure is passed on to the Bladder and Large Intestine for elimination. This function of separation works on the mental levels too, allowing us to sort things out in our minds in an effective way. If it's not working too well we can get easily confused and our vital energy becomes diminished as a result.

The Heart Protector has a particularly difficult role to play in today's world. This is because so much emphasis and investment is placed in our relationships and so much is expected of them and it's this function that takes the full force of the negative emotions if they go wrong. The joy of being alive gets thrown out of the window at these times. It is then left to the Heart Protector to deal with the fall out as it diverts negativity away from the Heart and then attempts to restore equilibrium once more to the person. It's secondary role is like that of an envoy or ambassador for the Emperor transmitting his commands throughout the Kingdom. By doing so, this Minister ensures that cohesion is maintained in the Empire through his contact with the people as he communicates the wishes of the Emperor, the core message being that they should experience peace and joy in their lives. Thus everyone knows what's going on and what is expected of them and any seeds of suspicion or conflict are laid to rest, thanks to this joyful mediator. In fact one of the acupuncture points on this meridian is actually called the 'Intermediary' and is used to bring a feeling of peace when there is emotional conflict within a person.

The Three Heater can be seen as a system of communication but different from that of the Heart Protector, neither of which have any parallel in Western Medicine. It circulates and warms the Qi energy in three sections of the body — the chest area, the area above the umbilicus and the area below it, thus connecting with all the major organs. Similar in concept to a central heating system, which circulates heat to different radiators around a house, it is responsible for the physical evenness of temperature in the body.

Just as a central heating system uses fluid to convey heat, so this Minister uses the warmed inner fluids to distribute this heat evenly thoughout the body.

It's emotional field of influence is in the outside world of a person whereas the Heart Protector's is with the inner one. Together they keep the equilibrium of the person intact, by acting like two well oiled gates that allow in what is good for the kingdom and filter out what is not. The Three Heater is also known as the Official of Balance and Harmony and is thus one meridian that is nearly always used at some stage during a course of treatment.

土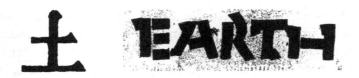

There is nothing which Heaven does not cover, and nothing which Earth does not sustain

Chuang Tse, 369 — 286 BCE Chinese Sage

The Earth Element

Acupuncture point names associated with this Element include: *People Welcome, Great Oneness, Abundant Splendour, Abdomen Knot, Encircling Glory Great Enveloping, Not at Ease.*

The Chinese saw the human being as a product of the marriage or fusing together of the powers of Heaven and Earth. The Heavens refer to the force that breathes life into us, together with all the cosmic influences affecting us from far away. The Earth refers to the Mothering force that provides us with all the nourishment we need, including our food and drink.

As "Mother Earth", you can imagine that this element has a lot to do with food and nourishment, both physical and emotional. The organs that are associated with the Earth Element are the Stomach and the Spleen. The Stomach receives all the food and drink that we take in and churns it around for some time, thus bringing it to a state where it can be effectively used by the Small Intestine. It is also responsible, together with the Spleen, for the whole journey down the oesophagus and into the Stomach itself.

In fact, the word 'stoma' actually means 'the mouth' and is seen as the Minister in charge of 'rotting and ripening' our food and drink. If the Stomach energy is out of balance, we can get physical symptoms like indigestion, belching, being overweight, ulcers, bowel problems and a lack of vitality. On the emotional level it can cause excessive worry within us. What it also does is enable us to digest, assimilate and absorb information and new ideas that come our way, each and every day and which is where the saying 'inwardly digest' comes from. So if our Stomach energy is out of balance, we may have difficulty taking in information that we see, hear or read; we'll not be able to mentally digest things so well. This can result in a muzzy head, poor concentration, inability to switch off, insomnia or obsessive preoccupation with things, especially food; in fact, we may use the words 'I can't Stomach it anymore', or 'I'm fed up to the teeth'.

The other organ associated with the Earth is the Spleen. Its ministerial function is likened to that of a Minister of Transportation as it has the responsibility of transporting food and drink throughout the whole of the digestive tract. Furthermore, it has been delegated the duty of transporting energy that has been derived from processing this food and drink to every corner of the Kingdom. It also filters damaged and dead cells out of the blood and helps to strengthen the immune system. If there is a problem there, we can experience symptoms such as poor circulation, heavy feelings in our limbs, problems with digestion and obesity as well as a lack of vitality.

On a mental level the Spleen is responsible for the processing and transportation of our thoughts, ideas and opinions. If it is not transporting things correctly we can experience symptoms such as poor memory, forgetfulness and obsessive thought patterns when we just can't shut off our minds. Feelings of being stuck in our lives, when we just can't seem able to move on, can also be a sign of an imbalance here, as is a craving for sympathy or a rejection of it.

A common cause of the Spleen becoming disturbed is the excessive consumption of refined sugars over a long period of time. So we should keep vigilant regarding our sugar intake which, in some people, can eventually lead to diabetes. Fibroids are generally associated with the Spleen because of its inability to move or transport energy, so you find that lumps of varying sorts can appear in the system. Obsessive collecting or hoarding of things, particularly the more bizarre, can also indicate an imbalance in the Spleen energy. But now, please fill in the fifteen part questionnaire that follows, which will give an indication of how your balance is, in respect of the Earth Element.

The following points will explain more about the Earth Element: how it can become unbalanced and how this will show in the symptoms. Being 'grounded' is to do with the Earth, and when we are it brings a feeling of stability and equilibrium within us. But if we become unearthed, perhaps as a result of a shock, moving house a lot, or travelling too frequently, we may experience a sort of inner insecurity. This can manifest as insomnia, excessive worry or a lack of nourishment, either physically or emotionally. Fecundity, fertility, an 'appetite for things', and Mother Earth are other key words that can be associated with this Element.

In the *Nei Jing* the Stomach and Spleen together are seen as being in charge of the 'storehouses and granaries' of the Kingdom which is an indication of the central role the Earth Element plays as a source of our fundamental nourishment. They also give us the ability to taste things clearly and because of its connection to Mother Earth, many problems associated with the menstrual cycle can arise through this Element being out of balance. It is a well-known fact that women who are undernourished, perhaps from an eating disorder, cease to have periods; but this can also happen when a person is undernourished emotionally. Irregular, or painful menstruation, excessive lethargy and irritability around this time are common symptoms of an Earth imbalance. However they can often be helped by Traditional Acupuncture, reflexology, herbal medicine and particularly nutritional advice. This latter therapy is not just about changing from white bread to organic wholemeal (although this in itself can be extremely beneficial) but encompasses a wide range of advice that allows our system to function more efficiently by giving it the nutrients it needs.

Self-Help Suggestions for Supporting the Earth Element

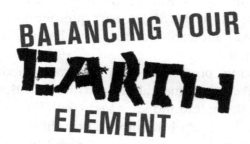

BALANCING YOUR EARTH ELEMENT

i) Regularity of eating is a very important aspect here. You should always try and have something for breakfast, lunch and dinner; organic porridge is a particularly good breakfast. The Stomach always works best when it has regular mealtimes.

ii) Try and cut down on red meats, pastries, oils, dairy produce, fats and, particularly, sweet things; too many of these foods deplete the Stomach and Spleen energies. Try and replace them with more fish, soya or rice milk, bio yoghurt and grains. Use extra virgin olive oil in preference to animal fats if you can.

iii) When you eat, try to do so in a calm environment or at least when you're not feeling stressed, as this helps the digestion.

iv) Try not to eat late at night because digesting food can cause insomnia.

v) Good pastimes for you would be walking, pottery and gardening, particularly growing vegetables (they all connect to the Earth).

vi) If you are troubled with unwanted, persistent, or obsessive thoughts, try the Bach Remedy White Chestnut. For those who tend to anticipate the worst happening, Red Chestnut is recommended.

vii) Tai Chi, Qi Gong and yoga are all excellent activities for you.

viii) Excessive work and thinking are not good for our Earth, particularly the Spleen energy, as they deplete it. Mental work is a lot more draining than physical work, so try and structure your working life better — a little more planning needed here.

ix) Foods that would be good for you would include aduki beans, apricots, dates, organic brown rice, ginger, parsley and cardamon.

x) Another good Bach Remedy for the Earth Element in general is Chicory.

xi) To gain perspective on the direction you'd like your life to go, particularly if you are feeling "stuck", Life-Coaching would be worth considering.

xii) You might experiment with Traditional healing music where the focus is on the Kung tone. It is recommended for nausea, digestive disorders, insomnia or excessive worry.

An Example of an Earth CF

Jill, aged 34, came with fertility issues. She and her partner had been trying for a baby for well over a year and tests had shown there was no obvious reason why she should not become pregnant. During the consultation she mentioned that she had, over the last two years or so, been drinking six to eight cans of fizzy, sweetened drinks a day and that for around the same length of time she had been energetically sluggish, particularly in the mornings.

The physical examination revealed that the pulse in her Umbilicus (belly button) through which the Conception Vessel meridian passes, was about one inch off centre, her tongue was heavily coated and her lower abdomen was very cold. Her voice had a singsong quality to it, her odour was fragrant and she had a noticeable yellow tinge on her face particularly around her mouth. After the diagnosis it was decided that her main energetic imbalance was in the Earth Element which was indicated by her facial colour, her predominant odour and voice quality, the coating on her tongue and the fact that her Stomach and Spleen pulses felt "soggy". This was caused by so much sugar in her drinks, and would also account for her lethargy in the mornings. Another important clue was that the reproductive area below her belly button was cold, which would further restrict her chances of becoming pregnant.

Treatment involved centering the Umbilical pulse, heating two acupuncture points on her lower abdomen on the Conception Vessel, meridian (some of whose points have a direct influence on fertility) with moxa and strengthening her Earth energy — specifically the Spleen meridian — using needle and moxa. She was also asked to remove the decorative piercing above her belly button because it was influencing an acupuncture point there and hindering the energy flowing through her Conception Vessel meridian. After a few weeks the point known as "the Door of Infants" which lies on the Kidney meridian, together with another called "the Gate of Life", situated between the Kidneys, were stimulated using needle and moxa.

Jill had also made great efforts from the start of treatment to cut out her fizzy drinks as well as dramatically reducing her chocolate intake and within three months she became pregnant. Early in the pregnancy, though, she suffered from morning sickness but this was eased using acupuncture together with wrist bands correctly placed on the acu points on her lower inner forearms.

She continued coming for treatment during the pregnancy for general support but also to help her relax as her job had, by this time, become very stressful. After a full term she gave birth to a healthy baby.

EARTH QUESTIONNAIRE

Below you will find 15 questions all of which relate in some way to this Element. Just read each one and give your immediate, honest answer. At the end we will see what your responses reveal about your relationship with the Earth Element.

1) **How do you like the colour yellow?**

   A. It's my favourite colour.
   B. It's O.K.
   C. It's my least favourite colour.

Yellow is the colour of the fields at harvest time in the late summer.

2) **How do you react if somebody shows you sympathy?**

   A. Always has a big effect on me — can even move me to tears.
   B. I quite like it when appropriate.
   C. Don't like it at all — can't handle it.

Sympathy or the inability to express it, is the emotion, together with worry, associated to the Earth Element.

3) **Do you like sweet things?**

   A. I find I crave them a lot of the time.
   B. They're fine every now and then.
   C. Don't like them — can make me feel a bit 'off' or head-achy.

4) **Do you like the late summer (Indian summer)?**

   A. I love it, it's my favourite season.
   B. I quite like it.
   C. It's my least favourite season.

5) **How is you relationship with your mother?**

   A. She's the most important person in my life by far.
   B. It's fine most of the time.
   C. It's always been very strained and difficult.

6) **Do you easily put on weight even though you don't seem to eat a lot?**

   A. Yes. Just by looking at food I seem to put on weight.
   B. I only put on weight if I eat too much of the wrong things and don't take enough exercise.
   C. I never put on weight even if I overeat.

7) **Are you a person who often gets obsessive about things?**

   A. Yes, very much so — particularly food and relationships.
   B. I can sometimes but really not often.
   C. No but I do love collecting things — it's one of my major hobbies.

8) **Do you like singing?**

   A. I love to sing.
   B. Yes, every now and then.
   C. I really don't like to sing and anyway I think I sound pretty awful.

9) **What is your best time of day?**

   A. Between 7 and 11 am GMT.
   B. No particular time.
   C. Not in the morning — it's my worst time, in fact I can feel lethargic a lot of the time.

These are the optimum times of the functioning of the Stomach and Spleen energies.

10) **Do you worry a lot and can this affect your sleep?**

   A. Yes — I feel I was born worried and often wake in the night churning things over in my mind.
   B. I feel I worry when it's appropriate.
   C. I hardly ever worry — I just shut it out.

11) **Do you get a lot of saliva in your mouth?**

   A. Yes a lot of the time.
   B. Only sometimes.
   C. I have the opposite — I get a dry mouth frequently.

12) **Do you get travel sick easily?**

   A. Not at all — in fact I'm needing to travel as often as I possibly can — can't get enough of it.
   B. Only very occasionally.
   C. Yes I do, and I never want to go on those rides at the fair either. They make me feel sick.

13) **How is your thinking ability compared to others?**

   A. I'm always sharp and quick in my thinking and in fact find it very difficult to slow my thoughts down.
   B. It seems OK.
   C. I'm generally very slow and easily forget things. I also find it hard to concentrate.

14) **Are you often troubled by nightmares?**

   A. Yes — I get them very frequently.
   B. Hardly ever.
   C. No, but I do dream a lot about empty houses and buildings in general. Yellow often comes into my dreams too.

15) **If you skip a meal can you feel a bit strange?**

   A. I always feel a bit light headed and get panicky if I can't get food when I'm hungry.
   B. Not really.
   C. I can go without food but I get Stomach cramps if I do.

Now add up your scores.

No. of A. answers.
No. of B. answers.
No. of C. answers.

Conclusions

IF YOU HAVE MAINLY B's: Your Earth looks in good shape. You have a nurturing personality without being over-protective, supportive without being too controlling. You are able to show sympathy at the right time and to the right degree without being either thick-skinned or too syrupy. Although you are considerate of others and concerned about their welfare, you are not one to worry excessively. You are likely to have a good memory and be able to concentrate effectively.

IF YOU HAVE MAINLY A's: It is an indication that the Earth energy is a tad over-active. This can manifest as a tendency to worry too much about things and as a result, becoming over protective, which in itself brings about feelings of insecurity. You may find yourself overly interested in food which can then lead to difficulties with your weight. Some people can put on weight just by looking at food and you might be one such person. Follow the recommendations for this Element and you will notice a difference sooner rather than later.

IF YOU HAVE MAINLY C's: It indicates a little weakness within the Earth. This may manifest with problems around food — feeling hungry but not able to decide what to eat for example. It's likely your energy is a bit depleted in general but particularly in the mornings. Your thinking can be rather scattered. You may find you can become rather too detached from other people, verging on the obsessional or conversely can get too preoccupied and absorbed in another person. If this is the case, then you may well benefit from therapies such as counselling or psychotherapy to help bring some perspective into your relationships. You may find it difficult to study and concentrate and to digest information; you might also feel a sense of being 'stuck' in your life. However, these are just signs of imbalances in the Earth Element and can be helped by the suggestions in this section.

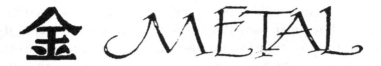

金 METAL

The Metal Element

Acupuncture point names associated with this Element include: *Heavenly Palace, Meridian Gutter, Very Great Abyss, Warm Current, Cloud Gate, Welcome Fragrance, Heavenly Vessel.*

The human being was seen in ancient times as a product of the fusing together of the powers of Heaven and Earth. In the *Nei Jing* the Yellow Emperor says "covered by Heaven and supported by Earth all creation in its most complete perfection is planned for its greatest achievement: humankind". Whereas the Earth is concerned with producing our energy from the nourishment provided by our food and drink, Metal is the Element that is responsible for receiving another form of energy — our breath. The Earth Element is seen as a female or Yin force, the Metal Element's connection is with the Father, in this case the Heavenly Father, and is a Yang force. So these two forces, the finite and the infinite, come together and create us — a being 4.54 billion years in the making!

This fundamental understanding of their relationship with the Universe was reflected in, of all things, their daily financial dealings. A traditional Chinese coin is round in appearance signifying the Heavens but with a square cut out of its centre which signifies the Earth. It was hoped that a reminder of the bigger picture of existence would have its positive bearing on this smaller, mundane side of it!

Confucius, the revered Chinese sage who lived between 551—479 BCE said this of mankind: *'Of all the creatures produced by Heaven and Earth, mankind is the noblest'*. It's difficult to recognize this fact sometimes but we all have that precious quality within us — it just needs to be uncovered from under the layers of dust we seem to accumulate and which over the years can grind our spirits down.

The two organs that are inextricably linked to the Metal Element are the Lungs and the Large Intestine. These have two quite different functions — one receives the pure air or breath from the Heavens, the other gets rid of the rubbish. On the one hand we have the most spiritual organ, the lungs, because of its connection with the infinite; whilst on the other hand we have the Large Intestine, which appears to have a very ordinary garbage disposal job of eliminating waste from our bodies. Even this Minister has a higher spiritual connotation because its ancient description tells us that it is responsible for "propagating the Right way of Living" — it rids us of what is no use and toxic to us and retains that which is of value. The latter may not sound as glamorous as the former but both are essential for our very survival.

There is a close connection between the lungs and our skin and in fact, because it breathes, the skin is called the 'third lung'. It has been said that the lungs contain around 300 billion minute blood vessels within them which, if laid end to end, would stretch for 1500 miles. If the lungs are in poor shape, problems can arise like eczema, psoriasis, acne, and skin rashes and a weakened immune system; we can also get respiratory problems such as asthma, bronchitis, emphysema or blocked sinuses. From the Large Intestine, if imbalanced, constipation, diarrhoea, lower abdominal pain, a poor sense of smell or too many rubbishy thoughts can arise. The Lungs are responsible for dispersing throughout our bodies a defensive form of energy

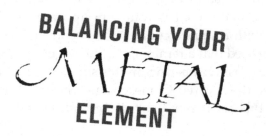

BALANCING YOUR
METAL
ELEMENT

called *Wei Qi* which flows just below the surface of the skin. This energy protects us from attack by outside climatic forces like wind, cold or damp which can cause infections such as colds, flu, sore throats or aching joints. It also shields us from psychic influences that can arise from excessive grief, sadness or gross disrespect that sometimes comes our way in life. If this *wei qi* is strong within us these things don't have such a debilitating effect on us, and we are more able to let them go and move on. This is why regular exercise, fresh air and preventive seasonal treatment at the beginning of Autumn is considered important as these help strengthen this *wei qi*.

Self-Help Suggestions to Support your Metal Element

i) If you are a smoker it would certainly help your lungs and Large Intestine, let alone anything else, if you were able to cut it out. If you enjoy smoking then there's no point, but if you sincerely want to stop, not just to cut down, then help is at hand. The two blocks to stopping are craving and habit, and of the two, craving is usually the more powerful. Ear acupuncture is very effective in dealing with the craving and allows you to cross the nicotine barrier smoothly without going up the wall. It's the craving that makes you feel like that. The habit side can generally be helped a lot through good hypnotherapy if that is troubling you. Both treatments on the same day can be very effective. So, if you can find that desire within you to stop, then go for it and don't start again.

ii) Rhythmic breathing exercises would be very good for you. Tai Chi, Qi Gong, yoga and meditation are all excellent for this.

iii) Foods that would be supportive for you are rice, peaches, onion, garlic and turnip. Also, those foods that contain high amounts of fibre could be very helpful too.

iv) If you tend to be very self-critical or hold your emotions in all the time, you might consider joining a positive thinking group (there is one in most towns), doing volunteer work, or joining the local ramblers club. Try not to be too perfect!

v) Foods to avoid would be milk, cheese, cream and pepper — replace with soya or rice milk, especially if you are prone to catarrh or sinus problems.

vi) To keep your skin tone in good shape and to allow the pores to be cleared and open, you would be advised to seek a qualified masseur. Skin brushing is another way of keeping the pores open, as are steam or sauna baths when appropriate.

vii) Placing yourself in situations or positions where spontaneity is demanded, as well as discipline, would be good for you. Paintball games, karate or fencing come to mind.

viii) Traditional Chinese healing music, incorporating the Shang tone theme, is effective in treating all types of respiratory diseases and can be helpful in cases of excessive grief or sadness.

ix) Star gazing would be a hobby to consider too as it brings us in contact with the awe-inspiring heavens.

x) Hill or mountain walking would be a good thing to get into as this helps strengthen the Lungs and thus our defensive energy whilst, at the same time, giving a broader perspective on life.

The following points will explain a little more about the Metal Element:

Of all the Elements, Metal reflects the quality and meanings in our lives. It is the shining jewels and rich ores that lie embedded within each one of us and we can feel these qualities in our skills and talents, our moral standards, our insights and deep spiritual feelings. On a more physical level Metal is to do with the ability to receive, to take things in as well as letting things go, which is what the lungs and Large Intestines do.

In the hierarchy of the Kingdom, the Lung's role is of a Chancellor or First Minister who relays orders from the Emperor to all the other Ministers, and thus is responsible for 'rhythmic order' within it. The Large Intestine's ministerial function is to 'initiate evolution and change' as well as having the added responsibility for all the roadways within the Kingdom — an essential ingredient for reducing traffic constipation!

Imbalances in these energies can produce a feeling of being cut off from other people and sometimes from ourselves too, causing an inability to receive the rich experiences of life that continually come our way. Because we cannot let go of our accumulated garbage we can become sort of poisoned on a mental/emotional level. This can result in feelings of bitterness, guilt, cynicism or suspicion.

By following the self-help suggestions we can start the process of rebalancing this part of us. Perhaps later on you might seek further help from therapies such as Traditional Acupuncture, shiatsu, homeopathy or hypnotherapy.

Incidentally, the current interest in body piercing, using various metals, should be viewed with some caution. For instance, there are over 100 points in the ear alone and care should be taken when selecting the area to be pierced. A common place for piercing on the body is in the umbilicus (belly button) in which lies the famous acupuncture point called *Spirit Deficiency*. It is one of the few points that are forbidden to needle and only Moxa (a heating herb) is allowed to be used there. The point just above it, another favourite for decorative piercing, is called the *Water Balancer* and is commonly used to treat conditions such as nephritis, oedema or hormonal imbalances. It would be most advisable to seek advice from an acupuncturist who would show you which areas are free of points so that your energetic system doesn't get disturbed.

Example of a Metal CF

Carol, 56, came with severe itching on her arms and upper torso together with a worsening of her sinus condition. She was also suffering from constipation, only going to the toilet once every three or four days. It transpired during the initial consultation that before these symptoms had become noticeable her elderly father had been taken ill and had subsequently died in hospital. Around the same time that this took place her husband became very unappreciative and cold towards her and as a consequence did not give her the support she needed at this difficult time. This resulted in her experiencing a great lack of self-worth and self-respect within herself and as a result she became quite depressed. Furthermore although she had been very close to her father she felt unable to grieve for him and shortly after his funeral began to suffer from this skin condition.

Her root imbalance was in her Metal Element which was indicated by the whitish colour around her mouth, her great difficulty in experiencing grief, and her voice which had a weeping quality to it. The Metal Element affects our ability to feel grief, has a bearing on our skin, lungs and Large Intestine and, if weakened, can result in a feeling of low self-esteem. Carol, because of this overwhelming stress, had produced a negative form of energy known as "aggressive energy" within herself. She might have been able to deal with her father's death without producing this but together with her husband's negative attitude towards her it had been the last straw.

The first treatment was to eliminate the negative energy from the system and subsequent treatments focussed mainly on her Lungs and Large Intestine meridians. Her pulses also revealed that she was energetically blocked in the area around her nose, between the Large Intestine and the Stomach meridians and when that block was removed , her sinus problems eased considerably.

After five further treatments her itching had reduced by around 50% and her bowels had become more regular. Furthermore she had been able to grieve for the first time for her father having experienced a dream early on in the course of treatment where her father had appeared to her in a way that consoled her. As a result she was able to let go of her pent up emotion, feel the grief and move on in her life which, as a consequence, reduced the itching even more.

Although the differences between her and her husband have not been rectified yet she has felt more confident in herself and has at least been able to face the situation with more clarity and strength.

THE METAL QUESTIONNAIRE

Below you will again find 15 questions. Just read each one and give your immediate, honest answer. At the end we will see what your responses reveal about your relationship with the Metal Element.

1) Do you like the colour white?

    A. It's my favourite colour by far.

    B. I quite like it.

    C. I don't like it at all — I'd never wear it.

2) How is your relationship with your father?

    A. We're extremely close — I don't know what I'd do without him.

    B. It's fine most of the time.

    C. It really hasn't been good — it's strained and difficult.

3) Is religion an important part of your life?

    A. I've always been a very religious person — I'd die for my beliefs.

    B. I do believe in a superior power.

    C. I don't believe in God — how could there be anything like that with so much grief around?

4) Do you like autumn time?

    A. It's my favourite season — I love it.

    B. I quite like it.

    C. It's my least favourite season and I always feel sad and melancholy at that time.

5) Which metal do you like to wear?

    A. I always love silver and wear a lot of it.

    B. I'm not bothered but if I do it's Gold.

    C. I don't like to have any metal next to my skin. It can make me itch.

6) **How is your sense of smell?**

    A. It's always very sharp — in fact too good.

    B. It's generally OK.

    C. Not good at all — I can hardly smell anything.

7) **Is being highly successful and having lots of money very important to you?**

    A. Yes — I'm always striving to get on and money is extremely important to me. It's a big status thing for me.

    B. I'm moderately into it.

    C. I'm not driven by money or success at all. There's no point — I'm happy to drift along.

8) **Are you the sort of person who has to do the correct thing all the time?**

    A. Yes — I love order and people say I'm a perfectionist.

    B. I like to do my best.

    C. I don't see the point in having everything just right — I'm happy to let things go on the way they're supposed to even if it ends up in a mess.

9) **Do you think discipline is important in life?**

    A. Yes I do. How else can people know their boundaries. Spare the rod and spoil the child is what I say. And that applies to adults too. People say I'm strict; I say I'm honest.

    B. I think some discipline is needed in life.

    C. I've had enough of discipline at school and at home to last me a lifetime. Who needs it — I'm hanging loose, man.

10) **Do you like ceremonial occasions?**

    A. Yes, I love to watch the military procession, changing the guard etc. I also like church rituals like baptisms and the marriage ceremony — they mean a lot to me.

    B. I quite like them.

    C. I don't think you need all that stuff — it's pointless to me.

11) **Do you have long-standing problems to do with your breathing?**

    A. I'm okay with my breathing but I do have problems with my bowels fairly frequently.

    B. It's generally OK.

    C. I've always been a bit tight-chested and prone to colds and bronchitis.

12) **Do you often have dreams of flying?**

    A. Yes, I get them quite frequently.

    B. Hardly ever.

    C. No, but I do have dreams where sorrow, grief, and the colour white come up a lot. Also I seem to be searching for something in them.

13) **How much does the emotion of grief have a part in your life?**

    A. I find I don't show much emotion at all. People say I'm stoical and cut off.

    B. I experience it every now and then.

    C. I feel grief a lot in my life — it seems to be my predominant emotion.

14) **What is the quality of your skin like?**

    A. I often get boils, eczema and dry skin.

    B. It's generally OK.

    C. I tend to have quite greasy skin.

15) **Do you have difficulty with authority in your life?**

    A. No — I like discipline and I respect authority and structure in life.

    B. I'm generally okay with it.

    C. I don't give a toss for authority — they can take a running jump for all I care.

Now add up your scores.

No. of A. answers.

No. of B. answers.

No. of C. answers.

Conclusions

IF YOU HAVE EIGHT A's OR OVER: Your Metal energy is a bit out of kilter. This can result in feeling cut off from people to a degree where you may feel isolated and, to others, appear unapproachable. You are a perfectionist and can hold yourself and others to the highest standards which is laudable until you become the slave of perfection, not the master. You are probably very successful but there is a price to be paid for this. You might need to be easier on yourself, trying not to be too 'perfect' and work on letting things go. Although you view other people's standards as inferior to yours, try to be less critical in your outlook. Make use of the self-help suggestions.

IF YOU HAVE MOSTLY B's: Your Metal Element is pretty balanced. Your life is well structured without being too rigid, you integrate well with other people although you find some of them rather slap-dash and undisciplined. You are honourable and self-controlled and respect authority and discretion. You can take in the richness of life when it's presented to you and are able to let go of things when their time is past. However, your friends sometimes think you a bit autocratic, distant and over-meticulous.

IF YOU HAVE MOSTLY C's: Your Metal energy is a little weakened. But remember with a little bit of change to your lifestyle, that special person that is you will be allowed to shine through.

For some reason (and a lot has to do with childhood and schooling) you perhaps experienced a lack of approval or recognition of your particular gifts and values, probably because you were not following the status quo: you rebel against authority and discipline — unfortunately a little too much. This is often accompanied with feelings of grief, loss and resignation as a result of this lack of recognition. Whereas those people with mostly A's need to loosen up a little, you would benefit by bringing a little more organisation and order into your life.

A trend with people who have a disturbance in this Element is a tendency to feel things very deeply. Because of this and the fact that they can feel disappointed or wounded if others don't recognise their depth of feeling they will either deny their existence or cover them up by appearing indifferent or nonchalant. To compensate for this they might strive to live a luxurious lifestyle, wearing expensive jewellery or driving a high quality car and focusing on earning a lot of money so that some sort of quality, at least, can be brought into their lives.

水 *water*

The Water Element

Acupuncture point names associated with this Element include: *Eyes Bright, Rich for the Vitals, Bubbling Spring, Door of Infants, Spirit Storehouse, Amidst Elegance, Wind Gate, Illuminated Sea.*

We now come to the fifth and last Element in the cycle of the Five Elements. This is the Water Element which is closely associated with the wintertime and is responsible for our will, our drive, our deep reserves of energy and our intellect. The two organs that are associated with this Element are the Bladder and the Kidneys.

In the Chinese view, the Kidneys are highly important because they contain our fundamental essence called *Jing*. This determines our basic constitution, or life's blueprint, governing our ability to grow from an embryo through all the different stages in our life. This is what our DNA appears to do and it could well be that our *Jing* and DNA (and even more complex codings that are currently coming to light), are very closely aligned. The Kidneys have a profound influence on our creative abilities because they store this *Jing*.

Within the kingdom of the human body we have, on the physical level, water in various forms — streams, rivers, reservoirs, lakes, springs and oceans. Around 65% to 70% of our body is made up of water and without its presence and availability everything dies. It appears so tranquil and serene when contained in a glass, but the power of it can move mountains and destroy towns and villages. It is an awesome part of nature because it has the power to give life and also to take it.

The Kidneys control all this water in the Kingdom whereas the Bladder controls the storage and distribution of water. We'll talk more about these functions after you've filled in the questionnaire.

Self-Help Suggestions to Support the Water Element

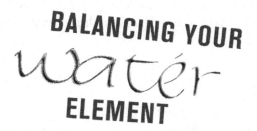

BALANCING YOUR water ELEMENT

i) For those who find it hard to relax, meditation, Tai Chi, yoga or hypnotherapy would all be excellent things to consider.

ii) Try and reduce your salt intake as this can have a negative effect on the Kidneys which, because they control the Heart (see Diagram 3, p. 12), has a knock-on effect there too. Unfortunately it is found in many foods, so choose well; certainly don't add it to your cooking. Also, try and reduce your consumption of cold drinks and raw foods, particularly in the colder months.

iii) If you are a person who experiences a lot of fear, phobias or paranoia you could well be helped by good hypnotherapy, psychotherapy or Traditional Acupuncture or by using one or more of the following Bach Flower Remedies: Rock Rose, Aspen, Mimulus, or Red Chestnut.

iv) In cold weather protect your ears (the cold enters here) and your lower back because this is where your Kidneys are situated and they can easily be affected by the cold.

v) If you are a tough, cold, detached, lonely type of person, try risking contact and attachment with others. If you find it all too difficult with human beings, you might find having a pet will be of benefit to you.

vi) Foods that would be beneficial to you would be: buckwheat, aduki and Kidney beans, kelp, red cabbage, water chestnuts, blueberries, cranberries and watermelons. Mussels, oysters, sardines, duck and pork would also be good. Try bringing miso and organic soya sauce into your diet. A good method of cooking would be the steaming method.

vii) Playing bridge, growing plants and flowers from seed or perhaps a water based sport would all be good pastimes to consider.

viii) During the winter months try and get to bed earlier and get up later as this helps to conserve our energy for the oncoming spring.

ix) Because your *Jing* is stored in your Kidneys and, for men, is lost during ejaculation, try and restrict the frequency to that recommended in the Fire Element section. It is important to keep to this frequency after the age of 50 and particularly so after 64.

x) Remember to be in a calm environment when eating whenever possible. Eating on the run is stressful, affects your digestion and puts strain on your system.

xi) Try traditional Chinese healing music incorporating the Yu tone. This resonates particularly well with the Kidney energy and is effective for anxiety, disturbed sleep and excessive fear.

xii) You might consider consulting a Five Element Feng Shui expert with regard to the most propitious layout of your house and also, if you have one, your garden. Proper advice in these areas can add to one's enjoyment of the house and garden, because the energy is allowed to flow more freely. Furthermore clutter gets eliminated, sleep quality can be enhanced and disharmony within the family unit can be reduced!

xiii) Few of us drink sufficient water, probably because it seems boring when compared to all the other drinks available. However water is the best thing for us and doesn't usually contain things like chemicals or sweeteners. It is recommended that we drink at least 1½ litres a day so you might find it more interesting if you add a squeeze of fresh lemon to a glass. Green tea is another drink to consider as it contains lots of vitamins and minerals, boosts the immune system, lowers cholesterol and slows down the ageing process! Its benefits were recognised and recorded in the *Book of Tea* written during the Tang Dynasty (618–905 CE) and is one of the most popular drinks in the world today.

One of the most important aspects of the Kidneys is that they store the *Jing* or essence of a person. All other energies of the body are dependent upon it. However, there are some aspects of our lifestyle that can use up this *Jing* rather too quickly. These are: overwork, too much stress, poor diet, excess worry, misuse of drugs, lack of sleep, excess alcohol and too much sex. We all would be well advised to conserve this storehouse of energy and guard it like the precious jewel that it is. If we do, then our overall health can only benefit and it will help to slow the ageing process down too.

In the organisational structure of the body the Kidneys are seen as the Minister in charge of all the water in the Kingdom. So if there is an imbalance here, symptoms like too much or too little urine, constipation, dry mouth (especially at night), night sweats and water retention can arise. They also govern the state of the bones and ears (the ears and the Kidneys have a similar size and shape), therefore brittle and soft bones as well as poor teeth and hearing problems can occur. Situations where there is a lack of flow in a person's life, coupled with rather too much anxiety and fear, can also be a result of an imbalance here.

The Bladder is seen as the Minister who controls the storage and distribution of water. It is the longest acupuncture energy pathway in the body with 67 points upon it. It starts near the corner of the eye, goes over the head, passing twice down the back and eventually to the little toe. Territorially it is by far the most influential of the 12 meridians and during its travels down the back it makes direct connections with all the other 11. This would help explain it's somewhat obscure description as being "like a governor of a province who is responsible for regions and cities".

The 67th point, named Extremity of Yin, is increasingly used these days by acupuncturists to help turn the unborn baby if it is in the breech position. Situations associated with this pathway include headaches, back pain, sciatica and painful knees, and because it controls the distribution of water, other symptoms that can arise are cystitis, incontinence and bed wetting. Furthermore, there can be low energy levels between 3 and 5 pm, which is High Tide time for the Bladder.

And finally, because the Water Element has a close connection to our bones, it would be good advice, in keeping with the spirit of preventive medicine, to get our structure checked out every now and then. In so doing any minor misalignments, particularly of the spine and the joints can be set right well before the problem becomes a major one. Just as acupuncture can help keep our energies balanced, so therapies like Physiotherapy, Osteopathy, Chiropractic or Bowen Technique can keep our structure balanced. Our structure and the meridian system are intrinsically linked so what we do to one affects the other and vice versa. In addition, these therapists will often give advice as to which exercises would be most beneficial in keeping the structure in good shape.

Example of a Water CF

Ahmed, who came from a strict religious background, was single and aged 22. He was training to be a male nurse and loved this work. His symptoms were a continual feeling of apprehension which drained him of his energy particularly in the late afternoon when he could hardly keep his eyes open. His sleep was poor and was troubled by vivid nightmares and he also had to get up a number of times in the night to pass water. He mentioned that he was worried about the needles and whether blood would be drawn during treatment. He was assured that only disposable, sterile, stainless steel needles were used and being so thin, no blood would be drawn.

The diagnosis was relatively straightforward in the fact that he had a slight bluish/black hue under and around the outer part of his eyes, his emotion was clearly dominated by fear, and his voice had a groaning quality to it which are all indications of a Water Causative Factor.

What was unusual were his pulses. Normally the amount of energy in the left hand pulses should be equal to or slightly stronger than those of the right hand side. In Ahmed's case, it was the opposite with the right hand set of pulses being stronger but also qualitatively more "hard" than those on the left. This pulse picture represents what is termed a "husband/wife imbalance" and is considered a serious imbalance in Five Element Acupuncture.

This observation made no sense to the practitioner at the time as the consultation had gone well with nothing untoward being presented by the patient and with good rapport having been made with him. Although he had sensed that his inappropriate emotion was one of excessive fear the practitioner still wasn't aware of the depth of it.

However, during the second visit, and with obvious difficulty, Ahmed was able to open up and tell the practitioner what really were his deepest issues. These were twofold. The first was that, some months ago, he had secretly converted from his own religion to another and should this fact be found out the consequences would be dire for him as he would be disowned by his family and friends. The other fear was that he had realised he was gay and had been unable to admit this fact to anyone close to him, not the least to himself. As he was the only male child in the family the situation was made even more difficult. He was thus caught in an unresolveable situation where he could neither go forward nor back. This had put an incredible strain on his mental and emotional state resulting in this severe imbalance arising in his system and revealed in his pulses. But at least it brought clarity to the practitioner's diagnosis who, with this understanding, was able to treat Ahmed for the "husband wife imbalance" and by doing so, avoided what could have eventually turned into a more serious illness.

The acupuncturist had to carry out this particular treatment three times because the patient would still be immersed in his problems on returning home and as a result, the imbalance would come back. After the third time of addressing this imbalance, and having focussed treatment in support of his Water Element, Ahmed gained enough confidence in himself to leave his family and to take up a similar position in another city which necessitated him moving out of his family home.

Although traumatic, it was the best solution for him at this stage and his life took on a much more positive and healthier direction after it. He continued to come for treatment sporadically and up to his most recent treatment this severe imbalance had not returned, he was much less tired and his levels of fear had reduced considerably.

WATER QUESTIONNAIRE

Below you will find the usual 15 questions. Just read each one and give your immediate, honest answer. At the end we will see what your responses reveal about your relationship with the Water Element.

1) **How do you like the colour blue?**

   A. It's always been my favourite colour.
   B. I quite like it.
   C. It's my least favourite colour — I'd never wear it.

2) **Do you like the taste of salty things?**

   A. Every now and then I find I crave it — especially when I'm tired.
   B. I quite like it every now and then.
   C. Yes I do; in fact I add salt to my food at nearly every meal.

3) **Do you like water?**

   A. Yes, I love swimming and would swim every day if I could — it's MY Element.
   B. It's OK.
   C. I don't like it at all — in fact I'm scared of it and l never go out of my depth.

4) **Are you a fearful sort of person?**

   A. People say I'm fearless. I find I seek out dangerous things to do whenever I can. I'm not scared of heights or deep water or scary movies.
   B. Only occasionally.
   C. Yes — I feel fear a lot and I'd never do anything that is remotely dangerous.

5) **When is your best or worst time of day?**

   A. My best time of day is between 3 and 7 pm GMT.
   B. I don't vary much in the day.
   C. I'm always very tired between 3 and 7 pm GMT — I always need a sleep then.

6) **How do you like the winter?**

   A. I love the cold, the bare trees and the short days — it's my favourite time of year.
   B. It's OK.
   C. I hate it — it's the worst time of year for me.

7) **Does water come into your dreams often?**

   A. Yes it does and sometimes tidal waves and the colour blue.
   B. Very rarely.
   C. No — but I often experience fear and cold in them.

8) **What condition is your head hair in?**

   A. Although I've still got plenty of hair it's in poor condition and I'm very grey for my age.
   B. It seems in good condition and I've plenty of it.
   C. I really don't have much hair at all. It's been thinning since my late twenties.

9) **Are you a very ambitious type of person?**

A. Yes, I'm driven to get on in life. I feel restless a lot of the time and people say I'm a workaholic and a survivor.
B. To some degree but it doesn't rule me.
C. I have no ambition at all. With my lack of vitality it's enough just to get up in the morning!

10) **How do you react to the cold?**

A. I thrive in it.
B. I can handle it pretty well.
C. I feel the cold goes through to my bones. I hate it.

11) **Do you feel very depleted after sexual activity?**

A. I am still very active and don't get drained very easily.
B. I'm OK if I don't overdo it.
C. Yes, particularly so now I'm in my forties. I think I might have overdone it when I was younger.

12) **How is the speed of your thinking compared to others?**

A. Even though I'm always on the go, my thinking is very electric — much quicker than others. I'm also very intuitive.
B. It feels average.
C. Because my vitality is low my thinking is very sluggish. Also I dry up if I have to speak in public.

13) **How are your waterworks at the moment?**

A. I pass a lot of water and have to get up in the night two or three times. I also frequently get cystitis.
B. They seem OK.
C. I don't think I go enough even though I drink a lot. It could explain my water retention problem and that may urine is not clear but quite coloured.

14) **Do you have problems with your teeth and gums?**

    A. My teeth are strong and I hardly have any fillings.

    B. They both seem OK.

    C. My teeth have always been problematic and most of them have fillings. My gums bleed quite frequently too.

15) **Do you like to be by yourself a lot of the time?**

    A. Yes, I'm much happier when I'm by myself and can look after myself, no problem. I don't feel lonely and like isolation and anonymity.

    B. I like to be by myself some of the time but then I'll enjoy company at other times.

    C. I get scared when I'm by myself. I don't like it and much prefer to be with lots of people.

Now add up your scores.

    No. of A. answers.

    No. of B. answers.

    No. of C. answers.

Conclusions

IF YOU HAVE MOSTLY A's: Your Water energy is a little imbalanced. You can be articulate, self-contained and clever with quite a lot of nervous energy and your close friends admire your intellect, intuition and electric thinking but they do feel you are rather tactless and suspicious. You are ambitious and fear very little, but you could do with offsetting your bluntness and detachment with tenderness and openness. Your character would benefit from some softening and it would be worth risking attachment or contact with others and a certain amount of social exposure to bring those hidden sides of you to the fore.

IF YOU HAVE MOSTLY B's: Your Water is pretty balanced. You are introspective without being withdrawn or detached, watchful without being suspicious. Your energy is quite even and you are careful without being fearful or hypochondriacal. You are curious about things and like to seek knowledge and understanding and are able to do many things in life without taking on undue stress. Your friends may think you a bit inaccessible emotionally and at times unforgiving, but generally you look in good shape.

IF YOU HAVE MOSTLY C's: Your Water is a little weakened. This is reflected in rather excessive anxiety and lowish energy levels, particularly in the late afternoon. You may dislike being alone and anonymous. Although experiencing fear protects us from dangerous situations you experience rather too much and tend to view life from this unnecessary perspective. You may also suffer from health problems to do with the spine, bones and ears. You can also suffer from a lack of willpower and can view other people and situations with a little too much suspicion. You may find yourself eating too many salty things to compensate for this imbalance within the Water Element. However, help is at hand. Please do use the self-help suggestions which have been proven to help with these sorts of imbalances.

How Diagnosis Works

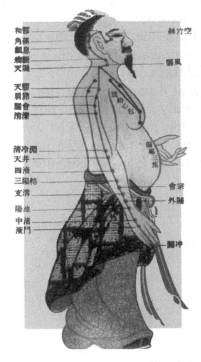

Figure 2   The Three Heater Meridian

The aim of diagnosis is to penetrate beyond the patient's symptoms to the core energetic imbalance that lies behind them.

Those who work with the Five Element system figure this out from a number of subtle signs exhibited by the patient. When one of the Elements is out of balance it will show in the Colour, Sound, Emotion and Odour of the patient. These are considered the four primary indications of an imbalance, the correspondences of which are shown in Diagram 2 (p. 10).

There are five Colours that can be seen on certain areas of the face when this occurs (see Diagram 8, below). These are green, red, yellow, white and blue/black and it's one of these that show up when a particular Element is in need of the most attention. Most acupuncture meridians flow through the face on either their primary or secondary pathways. This is one reason why the different colours are revealed there.

When you look at a person's face you may be unable to see these colours at first if you look too intently. Sometimes these colours, or more accurately hues, can best be seen at a glance or out of the corner of the eye. The second sign lies in the inappropriate sound, cadence or inflexion in the patients' voice, of which there

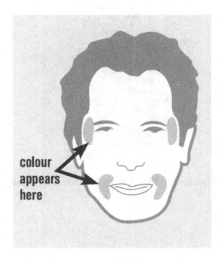

colour
appears
here

Diagram 8

Further five element correspondences

Element	Wood	Fire	Earth	Metal	Water
Balanced emotion	Assertive Confident Decisive	Emotionally well integrated. Able to move on after a broken hearted experience	Able to give & receive sympathy, support and nourishment	Able to feel loss & move on and to appreciate quality	Able to be appropriately cautious and to flow through life with confidence
Imbalanced emotion	Explosive anger Frustration Timidity Indecision	Over excitement Nervous giggling Lack of joy Vunerable	Obsessive worrying Craves sympathy or rejects it. Over protective	Absence or excess of grief Craves approval and recognition	Absence or excess of fear Constantly needs to feel safe
Nourishes	Sinews & tendons	Blood/blood vessels	Flesh	Skin	Bones
Expands into	Nails	Complexion	Lips	Body hair	Head hair & teeth
Sense organ	Eyes	Tongue	Mouth	Nose	Ears
Senses	Sight	Speech	Taste	Smell	Hearing
Body fluid	Tears	Sweat	Saliva	Mucous	Urine
Function of main organ	Ensures smooth flow of Qi energy	Houses the consciousness	Transforms & transports Qi	Governs Qi & respiration	Stores the essence (Jing). Controls water
Key words	Competitive, ambitious, active, practical. Can be domineering. Likes to be busy. Hates injustice. Should avoid the wind	Sensitive. Likes intimacy, comm-unication & excitement. Easily agitated & bored. Enthusiastic. Should avoid excess heat	Nurturing, loyal, harmonious. Likes to be included. Needy. Can be stubborn. Sympathetic and caring. Should avoid the damp	Likes order, cleanliness, structure & quality. Godliness. Needs to be right. Avoid dry climates	Honest, clever, self contained, strong willed, driven. Can be secretive and blunt. Ingenious and thrifty. Should avoid the cold
Highest expression	Compassion	Love	Empathy	Reverence	Wisdom
Confucian Virtue	Benevolence	Propriety	Faithfullness	Righteousness	Wisdom
Planet	Jupiter	Mars	Saturn	Venus	Mercury
Musical Note	Cheuh	Chiah	Kung	Shang	Yu

Diagram 9

are five types: shouting, laughing, singing, weeping and groaning. The third one is an in-appropriateness in one of the five emotions: anger, joy, sympathy/worry, grief and fear. The last and perhaps the most difficult to identify is one of the five odours emitted by the body, indicating which Element is struggling with a chronic imbalance. These are rancid, scorched, fragrant, pungent or putrid.

All this may seem rather esoteric or far-fetched but in fact some of these diagnostic observations were taught in certain medical schools in the Victorian era. Arthur Conan Doyle, who gave the world Sherlock Holmes, was himself a medical student and was strongly influenced by one of his tutors, a personal physician to Queen Victoria. He used some of these diagnostic methods of acute observation of the patient to astonishingly accurate effects.

Sometimes these signs stick out like a sore thumb and make the diagnosis relatively easy; at other times they are more difficult to perceive and then the work really starts for the practitioner! Every patient is like a detective novel, so to speak, and it's up to the practitioner to untangle and make sense of all these subtle signs so that the patient can be helped at the correct level of his or her disease. To do this effectively, and before anything else happens, the practitioner must leave his or her own worries and preoccupations outside the treatment room so that complete attention can be focused upon the patient. This effort, on behalf of the practitioner, which at times can be Herculean, helps bring about that unique relationship that must exist between practitioner and patient — one of trust, compassion and respect — for healing at a deep level to take place.

The 12 Pulses

The next important and fundamental tools in the diagnostic process are the 12 Chinese pulses.

Each of the 12 meridians has a pulse associated to it and their positions on the radial artery are shown in Diagram 10 (p. 111). They are the surface computer terminals of the body that give out information from deep within a person, which otherwise would be impossible to access even with today's advanced technology. The lighter or superficial pulse is felt with just a slight pressure on the wrist, whereas the deeper pulse is felt with a deeper pressure but still on the same position. Diagram 11 (p. 111) shows a physician from the Song Dynasty (960–1279 CE) with his fingers on these three positions which are, in fact, the same as those used in practice today. Diagram 10 (p. 111) shows a modern illustration of the positions and depth of the pulses that correspond to each of the 12 meridians. Thus you have three positions and two depths giving six pulses on each wrist, making a total of 12 in all. The pulses give the practitioner two things; firstly the volume or amount of energy in each of the organs and functions and secondly the quality of that energy, the latter being a bit more important than the former. Thus the practitioner will know if a

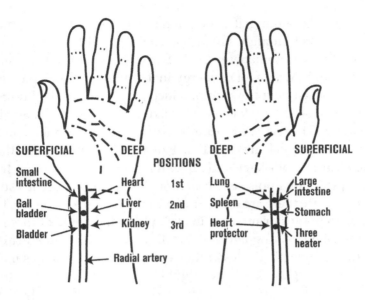

SUPERFICIAL	DEEP	POSITIONS	DEEP	SUPERFICIAL
Small intestine	Heart	1st	Lung	Large intestine
Gall bladder	Liver	2nd	Spleen	Stomach
Bladder	Kidney	3rd	Heart protector	Three heater
	Radial artery			

Diagram 10

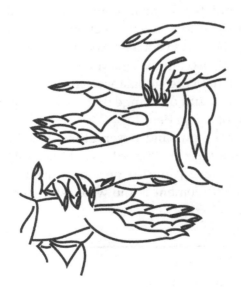

Diagram 11

meridian needs calming, if there is too much energy there, or energising, if there isn't enough. He or she can also tell from the pulses if there is a block in the energy flow. For example if the Liver energy feels full (that is, with a lot of energy in it) and the following meridian in the cycle (the one it flows into, which in this case is the Lungs (see Diagram 5, p. 14) is very low, then it's likely there is a block there in the Liver energy. The use of the appropriate acupuncture points on these two meridians, which are called the Exit and Entry points, can then be used to clear this blockage and allow the energy to flow more freely.

The quality of a pulse is more difficult to read because it's subtler, but also because there are more grades in the pulses to perceive. In fact there are 28 grades or nuances in each pulse and some of these have been described as long ago as 280 CE in the Chinese medical texts of the time. Some poetic descriptions of these pulse qualities include: "A pearl spinning in a dish" or "Tight like the string of a lute!" In general a quality in a pulse feels either confident and clearly defined (which is a positive sign), or thin and wiry (which indicates the need for attention). This aspect is usually dealt with first before any volume discrepancy is regulated. It can also give a deeper understanding of the state of an organ and a clue to whether treatment now would be appropriate in order to prevent a decline in its function in the future.

The pulses can also tell the practitioner if a treatment has been successful and if the core imbalance has been addressed. This is indicated by the amount of change that has taken place in the overall pulse picture of the patient.

There are other signs and observations that become apparent during the questioning of the patient at the initial consultation. These secondary signs can also provide invaluable assistance in working out which Element is the weakest in the energetic chain (see Diagram 9, p. 109).

Seasons

One of these signs is the way in which a person resonates with a particular season. This is because each season is associated with one of the five Elements and thus with a pair of organs or functions which explains why some of us feel better or worse at a particular time of year. The movements of the seasons also illustrate the cycle of the five Elements extremely well and, furthermore, upon each meridian lies a point whose effectiveness is heightened when used at the corresponding time of year.

From the quiet cold of the winter comes forth the dramatic birth of spring. Just as a drawn bow is poised to loose its arrow, so we too can feel the latent power of nature at this time as it bursts forth in such a dynamic way. It is the most eventful season of the year and one in which many of us experience a lot of upheaval. Just as in Nature, it kindles hope and excitement within us and creates the ability to look forward and make plans for the future. However if this energy, manifesting through the Liver and Gallbladder, is not firing on all cylinders then it can create a sense of feeling down and depressed, unable to see any purpose in anything, or a general lack of vision regarding the future. This can bring about feelings of anger, of being thwarted, or just generally being unsettled and depressed.

We then enter into the Summer time with all its associations with the Fire Element. This is when we can relax in the world enjoying the fullness, maturity and warmth of the longer days. It's a time for going out, communicating, meeting people and partying; a time when love is in the air. However, if our fire energy is impaired then maintaining those attributes associated with the Emperor (the Heart), like feeling in control, stable and compassion-ate, our ability to sort things out (as reflected in our Small Intestine energy), our evenness of temperature and our communication abilities (which are linked to the Three Heater) and our physical and emotional interactions (which are associated with the Heart Protector) will all feel like very hard work.

The next season in the cycle, the Late Summer, is that mellow time between the summer and the autumn when we reap the har-vest of our efforts put in during the year. The mellowness of this time of year brings about a feeling of equilibrium, of being able to rest in the palm of Nature's hand; a sense of being fulfilled. If an imbalance lies here in our Earth Element, some of us struggle to experience this sense of fulfilment and balance. We may feel like we are in a seasonal mid-life crisis and panic about what we haven't achieved, or that no one cares about us any more, or we long for the youthful days of Spring. At these times it's worth looking at the two Chinese characters that make up the word 'crisis'; one means danger the other means opportunity. Thus, out of each difficult situation that confronts us can arise a chance to learn from these experiences and an opportunity to move forward in our lives.

The Autumn, together with the Spring, is the time of the biggest changes in Nature, from the surge of Spring to the letting go of Autumn, which in turn is reflected in our physical bodies. For some of us this season can bring with it a feeling of sadness or melancholy, a precursor of the long nights of winter ahead. For others it's an exhilarating time, with the wonderful colours, the great movement of birds as they migrate, smells of woodsmoke and cosy evenings when the earth feels like it's being put to bed. Its being able to appreciate these changes and to accept them, rather than struggling against the natural flow, which is a lesson we all have to learn. Just as the Lungs take in and let go, so we too need to do the same. And just as the Large Intestine is responsible for "Change and Evolution" in the Kingdom, so we can strive to be in a place to embrace these changes rather than being afraid of them.

The last season in the cycle is the Winter; a time when the earth goes within itself as it contracts to adjust to the confines of the shortening days and the cold. Nature is at rest, plants return to seed and our reservoirs are slowly filled. We need to remember that there is a season for everything and this one calls out for the quiet storing and replenishing of our energies in preparation for the coming activity of Spring. In fact, the Kidney meridian, which together with the Bladder is associated with the Winter, has two points on it that convey this concept of storing; one is named the 'Spirit Storehouse' and the other simply 'The Storehouse'. They both refer to the storage of our deeper reservoirs of energy to be called upon when a person requires treatment at a more profound level.

By utilising the seasonal points contained within each meridian during the corresponding season of the year a person's energy can be synchronised with these cosmic movements. This in turn embraces the concept of preventive medicine, more details of which are given in the last chapter.

Colour

Another helpful sign gained from the patient is their preference for a colour, particularly if it is a strong preference to the exclusion of others. This is because each Element, and therefore its associated meridians, has a colour closely resonating with it which can give a clue to any imbalance lying within. Thus a strong preference for, or even a strong dislike of, a particular colour can reflect the state of our internal organs or functions, at least to some degree. These associations are shown in Diagram 2 (p. 10). Sometimes you find that a person's home has a strong one-colour theme in it, even down to the colour of the sheets and pillowcases, front door or car! They are all helpful diagnostic signs for the practitioner to work from.

Dreams

An additional tool in diagnosis is the understanding of a patient's dreams. Their interpretation has been used since ancient times in an attempt to get a handle on what is happening in a person's life or what might take place in the future. They are also used in a medical context as a way of assessing a person's current state of health. In the *Nei Jing* there are many references to dreams and their associations with the Elements. Practitioners today similarly gain valuable and profound insights into a person's Elemental balance from the content of a dream, particularly those that recur, are vivid or have a colour or elemental theme in them.

A dream can also help to confirm a diagnosis as well as to indicate how the healing process is progressing. They can also reveal the presence of more severe energy imbalances which, although rare, can prove invaluable to the practitioner as she or he strives to understand the nature of a patient's internal conflicts.

The following section gives associations that link to each of the Elements, together with some actual examples of dreams patients have had. In each the first part are examples taken from the *Nei Jing*, whilst the latter are observations and experiences of more modern dream therapy work.

Wood

- If the Liver energy is deficient dreams can include the presence of fragrant mushrooms, mountain forests, being engaged in fights and battles or of cutting one's own body.
- If the dream takes place in the Spring one can dream of lying under a tree without being able to get up — a sign of a deficiency or block in this Element.
- When the Gallbladder energy is deficient one can dream of fights, trials and suicide.

Modern Interpretation

- Struggling in making decisions or being unable to plan into the future.
- Futuristic dreams.
- Those where the colour green predominates.
- Where there are babies either being born or newly born.
- Those where there is an underlying feeling of anger.
- Where violence and blood occur.
- Where a person is being blown over by a powerful wind.

Example of a Wood Dream — James's Dream

The day after completing a contract of work I had the following dream: driving past a wood I saw a tree being cut down because it was dead. Then, next to it, appeared another tree, of the same species except that this one was full of life. It was tall with lush green leaves and with bunches of blue/black fruit growing abundantly upon it.

Explanation

In James's dream there is a strong Wood association reflected in the letting go of one part of his life that had served its time and was no longer able to influence his future life, and the birth of a new dimension. (At this time James was waiting for an interview for what he considered would be a perfect job for him.) In its place, as good fortune would have it, a new growth had taken place, which, being of the same species is substituting what has become old with something new. As this tree is tall it would indicate that the type of job was being nurtured within his mind for some time. And because of the Wood Element's association with good planning and the ability to look ahead in the mind's eye, it would give the practitioner useful diagnostic information as to the healthy state of his Wood Element. Furthermore, Wood being the product or child of the previous Element Water, whose associated colour is Blue/Black, would thus be seen as another positive reflection of his internal energy flow. The fact that the tree bore fruit, and abundant at that, would again be seen as very positive. On another level this would be an indication that the new job James was going for would be right for him. Because this episode took place in the Spring the treatment that was given was the needling of the seasonal points on both the Liver and Gallbladder. These points emphasise the Element's positive characteristics, particularly of the Liver, whose point name is 'Great Esteem', and would go with the flow that was taking place in James's life at that time. (James did in fact land the job and it did prove to be what he wanted.)

Fire

- If the Heart energy is deficient, its spirit won't be contained within it and will 'float' at night causing insomnia, disturbed sleep or excessive dreaming.
- When this Element is deficient, one dreams of fires, of being rescued from fires, of volcanic eruptions, of hills and mountains; particularly when they take place in the Summer.
- Dreams of towns or cities filled with people or of main roads can be indicative of an imbalance in the Small Intestine function.

Modern Interpretation

- Most sexual dreams are associated with the Fire Element, particularly the Heart Protector, and the Three Heater officials.
- Those that regularly contain feelings of emotional vulnerability, confusion or being overheated are often a sign of a disturbance in the Fire Element.
- Those dreams with a strong red colour in them.
- Those where there are throngs of people milling around but no one is taking notice of the person having the dream.
- Those where there feels to be a struggle in sorting problems out and where nothing in the dream gets accomplished.

Earth

- Dreams where there is a lack of food and drink in them.
- Those where buildings and walls are being put up.
- Those where chanting, and playing of music occur; when the body feels heavy and where a person experiences difficulty in getting up.
- The appearance of hills, marshes, ruined buildings and storms can indicate a disturbance in this Element.

- If the Spleen is deficient one can dream of being hungry, and if it takes place in the late Summer one can dream of building houses. If it is in excess, one can dream of singing and feeling very heavy or of abysses in mountain areas.

Modern Interpretation

- Earthquakes and nightmares are classic signs of Earth-related problems.
- As are relationships with one's Mother, sweet things, singing and feeling like one is stuck in a quagmire, hardly able to pull one's self out.
- Dreams where the colour yellow is predominant.
- Dreams that contains rooms or buildings, particularly those relating to houses.

An Example of an Earth Dream

In Caroline's dream, she enters a large, old house, which feels familiar to her. Her Mother is in the house, the walls of which are painted in various shades of yellow. She senses she is coming home, but feels stuck somehow and her legs, whilst walking towards her Mother, feel as though they are in quicksand. She struggles on but can't reach her Mother who reaches out to her, but Caroline is unable to grasp her hand to be pulled out of the mud.

Explanation

In this example, there is a very clear Earth connection, indicated by the presence of a house, the colour yellow, the Mother figure, quicksand and being stuck. The Earth Element governs two organs — the Stomach and Spleen — and the fact that Caroline feels stuck and unable to move forward points more to the Spleen energy being the one most in need of attention. This is because the Spleen is seen as the Minister in charge of Transportation in the kingdom and in this case appears to be under-active. This would indicate the need for an energising treatment rather than a calming one. Of the 21 points on the Spleen meridian, the most appropriate of them that come to mind to use at this stage of treatment is Spleen 8 whose name is the 'Earth Motivator'. The effect of this point is to move the energy forward when it has become sluggish.

During treatment Caroline had expressed how there had been difficulties in the relationship with her Mother when she was in her teens. This had culminated in her sudden and dramatic departure from home, which left her Mother devastated. Since treatment Caroline has been more inclined to re-open dialogue with her Mother and, provided she can be allowed reasonable freedom in her life, there is every chance that this relationship can be re-established.

Metal

- Those dreams in which white objects appear.
- Where one is frightened, cries out or soars through the air or sees strange objects made of metal.
- Dreams where fields and landscapes appear often relate to the functioning of the Large Intestine.

Modern Interpretation

- Flying dreams and aeroplane crashes.
- Those involving swords or metal weapons in general.
- The Father figure, searching for something, being lost, feelings of grief and weeping are all associated with the Metal Element.
- Those dreams with a predominantly white colour in them.
- Those where the theme is of garbage and rubbish.

Water

- Dreams of ships, boats, and people drowning or lying in water and being frightened. The sensation of the back and waist being split apart.
- Approaching a ravine, plunging into water, or being in water.
- When the Kidneys are deficient one dreams of swimming in water after being shipwrecked.
- If a dream takes place in winter, when one is plunged into water and feeling scared, is also an indication of a disturbance in the Water Element.
- When the Kidneys are in excess one dreams that the spine is detached from the body.
- When the Bladder is deficient one dreams of taking walks and excursions.

Modern Interpretation

- Tidal waves occurring in dreams often indicate a disturbance in this Element.
- Being frozen, sexually frigid, fearful and the winter time are all themes that indicate a connection to the Water Element.
- Those where the colour blue/black predominates.
- Those that contain images of subterranean streams or underground reservoirs.
- Those where the moon phase regularly appears, particularly the full moon which, because of its affect on water, can indicate a disturbance within this Element.

There are other types of dreams that can indicate a more severe imbalance or block within a person. These fall into three categories and are commonly revealed in the following types of dreams. It should be noted, however, that these forms of blocks are rare, particularly those in categories 2 and 3.

Category 1

- The presence of polluted or dirty water, or where garbage or dead bodies are floating in water.
- Where trees or vegetation are being cut down by metal implements.
- Where water is extinguishing fire.
- Where fire is melting metal or metal objects.
- Where trees and vegetation are unable to keep the earth together and it becomes rapidly eroded.
- Where earth is damming or soaking up water.
- Where there is a presence of derelict and dark houses.
- Where there is a presence of snakes or rats.
- Those where there is an aggressive black dog in them.

Category 2

- Where there is a sense of an evil presence in the dreams.
- Where there is a presence of ghosts, monsters or scaly insects.
- When there is a feeling of being controlled by another person or by a malignant external force or power.
- Where one is feeling controlled by some dark inner force.

Category 3

- Where a person feels they are being pulled apart, either physically or emotionally.
- Dreams that contain a feeling of immense conflict within a person. This can include conflict within one's family, or where the sexual or personal identity of a person is struggling to survive, be recognised or understood.
- Where there is a feeling of complete resignation or extreme fear.

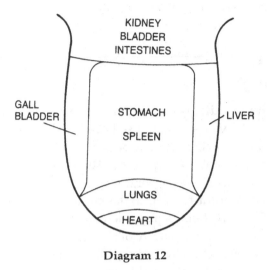

KIDNEY
BLADDER
INTESTINES

GALL
BLADDER

STOMACH

LIVER

SPLEEN

LUNGS

HEART

Diagram 12

Furnished with these indications of more severe blocks the practitioner will be directed to one of three different treatment protocols that are required to address each of these conditions.

Tongue Diagnosis

This is another one of those kind gifts provided by Nature to those interested in an external reflection of an internal disturbance.

Certain sectors of the tongue correspond to the organs and it is the understanding of these areas together with their colour, markings, shape and coverings that give a clue to the inner state of the organs themselves. Diagram 12 (above) shows these areas.

Sometimes the sides of the tongue can appear indented which is often a reflection of the state of the Spleen. A groove down the middle can point to a possible disturbance in the Heart energy whilst a thick white coating over the whole of the tongue generally indicate a problem with the Stomach. Often when a person tidies up their diet, by cutting out junk food and drink, their tongue covering becomes normalised indicating that the Stomach, as least, is benefiting from an easing of the onerous task of dealing with those toxins.

Face Reading

Another method of diagnosis, which has been used by physicians for well over 2,000 years, is Chinese Face Reading or Physiognomy. The health and constitution of a person is often reflected in their physical characteristics, particularly the lines, indentations and markings on the face. Thus a person with two deep clefts between the eyebrows can point to an imbalance in the Wood Element particularly the Liver. If there is just one cleft there it is often a sign of a disturbance in the Earth, usually of the Stomach energy. Horizontal lines across the forehead can indicate an excessive intake of sugar, fats and liquid, whereas vertical lines are indications of too much animal fats or an excessive intake of salt. A horizontal line above the upper lip can indicate menstrual or ovarian problems in women and sometimes sexual difficulties in both men and women. This sign is usually understood as reflecting the state of the Earth Element, particularly of the Spleen.

The lips are seen as corresponding to the Earth Element, particularly the Spleen. If the lips are swollen it can indicate some disturbance there. The corners of the mouth correspond to the Duodenum (the entrance into the intestine) and a cyst there can indicate a problem in that area. If the area underneath the eyes is a little puffy or of a darker colour than the rest of the face, this can be a sign of a disturbance in the Kidney energy.

Miscellaneous

- The state of the nails is a useful reflection of a person's inner health. Nail problems can indicate a nutritional deficiency, such as a lack of calcium, zinc, or vitamin B2, due to poor diet or digestive problems, which inhibit the absorption of nutrients from our food. In Chinese medicine the nails reflect the state of the Wood Element, particularly the Liver, as they rely on its energy to store the blood, which then nourishes them and keeps them moist. So if the nails are ridged, dry, discoloured or brittle it can suggest that there is a problem in this area.

- The state of the functioning of the Three Heater can be gauged using a simple test. Place your hand palm down on your chest area against the skin, then above the belly button and lastly just below it. All three areas should be of equal temperature, but if one is either much hotter or much cooler than the others then there is likely to be an imbalance here. However this can usually be regulated using Traditional Acupuncture.
- If the toe that is next to the big toe is somewhat longer, this can indicate a disturbance in the Earth energy, particularly of the Stomach.

One other important area to which practitioners attach great importance is the childhood experiences of the patient. For many it was generally a happy time, even idyllic, but for some their experiences of this time will have laid down imbalances in one or more of the Elements. For instance if a child had parents who were continually overbearing or controlling, or if there was anger and violence either shown to the child or between the parents, this will have caused a disturbance within the Wood Element, particularly the Liver. If a child was constantly denied love and affection, or if there had been an emotional split within the family unit at this time it is likely that the Fire Element would become disturbed. Similarly, if a child was never shown understanding or was denied nurturing, particularly from the Mother, or if there were a number of house or country moves at this time these factors would, to some degree, have disturbed the Earth Element. The Metal becomes imbalanced if the child was expected to be perfect or to gain unrealistically high achievements in their life, or where authority either from parents, teachers or religion was constantly hammered into the child. And lastly an atmosphere of fear, isolation, suspicion or sarcasm would cause a disturbance in the Water Element within a person.

Armed with these insights, the practitioner would aim to restore order and balance to those Elements within a person which have become disturbed from that time and which, even years later, still affect the now grown up child.

The Five Element Acupuncture Consultation

What Happens When I First go for a Five Element Acupuncture Consultation and Treatment

Your first visit should last around one to one and a half hours and this consultation will form the basis for future treatments. From the information you give your practitioner together with the observations made during the questioning and from the physical diagnosis, will enable them to figure out a treatment plan for you. This is aimed at relieving not only your symptoms but also tailoring it to address you as a unique individual.

It would be very helpful if you could bring to the consultation a short medical history going back to early childhood, if possible, together with a list of any medication that you are presently taking. It would also help if you could refrain from wearing perfume or aftershave. The initial visit will usually be divided into two parts.

The first part will consist of questions put to you by your practitioner and these are likely to include:

- Why have you come for treatment? (Some people come for preventive treatment and may not have any noticeable symptoms.)
- Details of your main symptoms e.g. how long have you had them?
- What makes them worse?

- Are there any secondary symptoms that you are experiencing?
- The state of your parents health. (This can give a clue as to which illnesses tend to run in the family.)
- Your birth. Any trauma experienced at this time? (For some practitioners the exact timing of your birth would be helpful.)
- Your medical history including past illnesses, accidents, injuries, or operations.
- What significant events were there during your childhood e.g. did you move house often? How were your relationships with your parents and siblings? Any illnesses at this time? Your experiences of school? Did you experience bullying at this stage?
- Significant events during your teenage years.
- Your job — do you enjoy it? Is it a burden to you?
- The quality of your sleep and any noticeable dream patterns?
- Your appetite, favourite foods, or any reactions to certain foods?
- What sort of things do you drink during the day?
- Do you feel thirsty a lot of the time?
- Your alcohol intake, if any. How does it affect you?
- Do you smoke? If so, how many?
- The state of your bowels and waterworks.
- The state and condition of your eyes, ears, nose, teeth and mouth.
- Your levels of energy throughout the day.
- Do you suffer from headaches or migraines and what form can these take?
- How is your bodily thermostat, heat balance, pattern of perspiration and circulation?
- How is your weight? e.g. does it noticeably fluctuate?
- Do you bruise easily?
- For women — information on the period cycle, pregnancies or the menopause and condition of the breasts.
- Some practitioners will ask for your favourite colour, season, time of day and climactic preference e.g. how do you react to wind, heat, humidity or cold?

Other miscellaneous questions might include:

- Do you suffer from travel sickness?
- How do you respond to injustice?
- How you respond if sympathy is shown to you?
- How do you feel in intimate social situations?
- Do you find it a struggle to make up your mind about things?
- Can you make plans for the future reasonably well or is this a difficult area for you?
- How is the state of your emotional balance at present — for instance, does anger, fear, sadness or grief hold you to ransom at times?

There may be other questions put to you but these cover the majority of them.

You will then move on to the second part — the **Physical Examination**.

This will always include the reading of the 12 pulses, six on each wrist. Others can include:

- palpation of the abdomen
- taking your blood pressure
- examination of your tongue
- assessing the position of your umbilical pulse
- observation of the state of your nails
- noting any scars you may have
- checking the heat (or lack of it) on your upper chest, the area above your umbilicus and also below it.

Some practitioners may carry out what is termed an "Akabane" test which assesses the bilateral balance of energy in the 12 meridians using a glowing thin taper held close to your fingers and toes (not painful!). Five Element practitioners, during the course of the diagnostic process, will observe the colour on your face, the sound of your voice, one of the five subtle odours we all have, and how your emotional balance is at this time in your life — is there one that appears to be inappropriate?

You might also be asked questions regarding your structure, neck, spine and joints.

All this information is of great importance to the practitioner, simply because it helps pinpoint the area or Element most in need of support. Some of these questions may appear rather intrusive for some people, but it is done solely that the practitioner may help you in the most effective and efficient manner. It goes without saying that all information given is **totally confidential**.

By now, furnished with this information you have provided and together with the observations made, the practitioner may have formed an idea of the state of your energy balance. They might also have determined where the root cause lies within your system which for the 5 Element practitioner is the one Element of the five most in need of support. However, it can take two or three more visits before that becomes clear, sometimes even longer. All these questions, together with the observations, have a direct bearing on understanding the state of your internal energy balance which is why the training, commitment and experience of the practitioner is so vital.

Sometimes during the consultation or subsequent treatments the patient may come out with what is termed "a Golden Key". This is a flash reaction initiated by the patient and captured by the practitioner's experience and intuition. It may be a throw-away gesture, a passing remark, a facial expression or surge of colour on the face when talking about something that is of great importance to them: or it may be something that doesn't quite make sense to the practitioner or that strikes them as odd. It can be the realisation of a dream, an emotional experience or incident that surges up in the patient's memory. These can allow the practitioner's perception to penetrate and understand what lies at the core of the patient's life experience and which may have produced an imbalance in one of the Five Elements.

Locked away in our memory are all those influential experiences, particularly from childhood, which have brought us to where we are today, at least to some degree. Some of those experiences would have caused a patient's imbalance which they may have completely forgotten about, and often the diagnostic process can allow these insights to be revealed and understood.

This can even go back as far as our own birth. In my own case it was during the birth process when forceps delivery became necessary. In those days, in the 1940s, this procedure was not as sophisticated as it is today and the forceps used then caused a severe disturbance both on the muscular functioning and also on the pathway of the Small Intestine meridian which passes through the neck, across the face and up to the ear. However, nature compensates, and allows us to forget many unpleasant things that have happened to us although the reverberations still remain within us.

All this may sound a bit unsettling but, in fact, remembering things that once deeply affected us, but which have been pushed to the back of our minds, can bring forth much emotional freeing up which in itself can constitute an effective treatment. It can also bring about an understanding of the patterns that have caused certain things to happen in our life and how we can best avoid them in the future: this is how valuable the consultation process can prove to be.

Depending on how long the diagnostic process has taken (my longest was over 2½ hours) will determine what then follows. If it has been straightforward the practitioner may then carry out a simple rebalancing treatment. If it has been more complicated they may want time to consider all the information that has been presented to them before carrying out a treatment which in this case will be on the next visit.

Treatment is usually once, sometimes twice, a week to begin with. However, as soon as the practitioner feels she or he is working on the correct root cause and the patient starts to feel better and the symptoms recede then this moves on to around once a fortnight. If all continues going to plan, this extends to once every three or four weeks or so and eventually to around five times a year at the change of the seasons in order to maintain an optimum level of health. Alternatively the patient may want to resume treatment when the need arises for them as it is always up to the patient to have the last word in this matter.

It is usually advised that a patient should take it easy after treatment, if possible, and refrain from consuming alcohol or fatty foods during the rest of the day.

Most professional acupuncturists are recognised by some private health insurers these days. Many reimburse all or part of the cost of treatment. These include: BUPA, AXA-PPP, Healthshield, Simply Health, Sovereign Health Care and Westfield, etc.

Natures differ, and needs with them, hence the wise men of old did not lay down one measure for all.

Chuang Tse, 369 — 286 BCE Chinese Sage

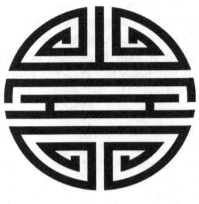

Longevity

How Acupuncture Works

In a nutshell, illness or disease is seen as an imbalance in the Qi energy of a person. This occurs when there is too much energy, too little, or a block in its flow. Very occasionally it is to do with the presence of destructive energy within the system.

Acupuncture's role is to assist nature by influencing the energy in such a way that it returns to its natural flow and balance. This is achieved by inserting very fine sterile disposable needles into one or more of the acupuncture points or heating them with a herb called Moxa, in a process called Moxibustion. The Chinese word for acupuncture is *zhenjiu* — *zhen* means needle and *jiu* means heating herb or moxa and both are often used together in treatment.

Although Moxibustion in recent years has been overshadowed by the use of needles, it is itself an invaluable therapy. It is effective in the treatment of chronic disorders, conditions of deficiency, and those aggravated by the climate, particularly cold and damp, both of which are prevalent in Northern Europe. When used together with needles, which has been the case for centuries, they produce an awesome combination. The energising, drying and warming properties of Moxa on the skin combine wonderfully well with the effects of needling which regulates the Qi energy within the patient.

Most acupuncture points can be moxa'd and needled with the exception of a small number which are forbidden for safety reasons; there are also a few that are forbidden during pregnancy but all properly qualified Acupuncturists will know of these point restrictions. Moxa can be applied in various ways — the most common method being the use of a small amount of the herb rolled

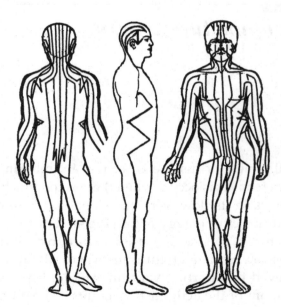

Diagram 13

into a ball about the size of a small pea. It is placed directly on the skin above the point and lit which then smoulders down so that an impulse of heat is transferred to the point. It is removed quickly so that it doesn't scar the skin and the common numbers used on a point are between 3–5 although there are some that can take a lot more.

Another way to apply Moxa is using a Moxa stick which looks like a cigar and which, when lit and glowing, can pump a lot of heat into the system over a much wider area than the pea-sized method. Moxa, whose Latin name is Artemesia Vulgaris and which is similar to Mugwort, a common herb in Europe, has a unique built-in power to project the wonderfully pleasant heat that it produces deep into the system. Most people love the warm sensation and, although the smell is pungent, many patients love that too, although these days smokeless Moxa is also available.

A third method is where an amount around the size of a child's marble is clamped to the head of a needle, after being placed in the required point. When it is lit and glowing, it transmits the warmth down into the surrounding area. This method is often used where there are tight or cold muscles, for example "frozen shoulder", or for hip problems, which can benefit from this more direct and deeper approach.

The term Moxa is derived from the Japanese, Moe kusa, which literally means "heating herb". Although its use probably predates that of the needle, the first books written about it only appeared around the 3rd century CE. There was one monograph, written in 1128 CE, which concentrated on the effects of just one famous point called "Rich for the Vitals" that is located either side of the upper spine. It was used then, and still is today, for longstanding chronic problems and is one point that can be moxa'd up to 50 times in one treatment.

Moxa is also useful for those patients who are afraid of needles, for younger children and for older patients to strengthen their immune system and help them to cope better as their vitality diminishes.

By choosing the appropriate point and with the correct manipulation of the needle, the Acupuncturist can bring Qi to a weakened meridian, disperse it from where it is too full, or unblock it.

There are 12 main meridians that govern the ten organs and two functions whose pathways are showed in Diagram 13 (p. 134). They connect to their corresponding organ via a deeper pathway. Additionally there are two others which, although not corresponding directly to any organ, act as a sort of energetic reservoir for them particularly in times of stress. They are named the Conception Vessel which runs up the front of the body and the Governor Vessel which runs up the back.

Classically, there are around 365 points, although the number within each meridian can be different. For instance, the Heart meridian has nine points , the Bladder 67, the Stomach 45 and the Spleen 21 etc. The size of an acupoint is small and has been described historically as being the size of an uncooked grain of rice. The general feeling these days is that they are smaller even than this which is why a point can sometimes be missed on the first attempt even by experienced practitioners. Each point has a name and, whilst some have lost their meaning in translation, others give the practitioner a deeper understanding of the inherent effect of that point e.g. Bright and Clear (Gallbladder 37), Abundant Splendour (Stomach 40), Door of Infants (Kidney 13), Heavenly Palace (lung 3), Spirit Gate (Heart 7), Bubbling Spring (Kidney 1) and Happy Calm (Liver 3) etc. Furthermore, each point has a unique action built into it which is subtly different from all the others. Some have more of a bearing on the physical aspect of the patient, others on the emotional levels and some on the deeper levels. Understanding these different potentials inherent in each point is fundamental to the practice of Traditional Acupuncture; equally important is the appreciation of and respect for them. This respect is gained partly from the extensive training process, partly from the practitioner's own experience and intent, and partly from their focus during the act of needling. Some sensitive patients are intuitively aware of this latter attribute during treatment. I once had a patient who, after I had needled a point on him, said to me, "you weren't there, were you?". He was right; my mind had wandered off somewhere just at the critical moment of needling and I wasn't "present" and he knew it! By being focussed the practitioner can better act as an instrument and thus can help transmit more effectively the unique quality of the point to the benefit of the patient.

The depth of the points vary considerably but most of them lie between 1/10" to 1" below the surface of the skin. Although there are points over the whole of the body the vast majority, and the ones that control the energy and which are used most of the time, lie below the elbow or below the knee. Those that use the Five Element system of acupuncture tend to use only a few needles — commonly between 4 and 8 and occasionally only one. The main exception to this rule is for a treatment known as 'draining aggressive energy', when polluted energy is removed from the system using a total of 12 needles lightly placed either side of the spine.

Because the needles are so thin — about the width of a hair or two — no blood is drawn during treatment. When a point is touched you feel a slight dull, achy, cramping, tingling sensation which really is no big ordeal. They are either left in place for a time or are in and out in a second.

It is worth mentioning here once more that there are three types of acupuncture. One category treats symptoms like back, shoulder, joint and sciatic pains. The second is called Western Medical Acupuncture which requires more training and treats some of the conditions you go to your doctor for.

The other, known as the Traditional or Classical approach, treats each person as a unique individual and seeks to address the root cause of the problem and demands by far the most rigorous training of them all. In this style no two patients are treated the same, even if their symptoms appear identical. A quote from the philosopher Chuang Tse (4th century BCE.), encapsulates this idea well: *'Natures differ, and needs with them, hence the wise men of old did not lay down one measure for all'*.

This latter approach is particularly helpful for problems that have been around for a long time or for those that arise more from an emotional disturbance within a person. The key point about the emotions is this: we shouldn't get locked into them for too long because if we do problems can arise in the meridian to which that emotion corresponds (see Diagram 2, p. 10). The idea is that we return to a reasonable state of equilibrium fairly soon after the storm of that emotion has passed and this style can help facilitate this process. Furthermore, because it treats the patient rather than the symptoms, it is very effective for those who come with a wide variety of seemingly unrelated problems but which, in fact, stem from the same root cause. Additionally it can deal with those cases where there are indications of more serious or life-threatening energy imbalances.

To give you an idea of the sort of things people can come with for this type of treatment, the following list provides a glimpse of its varied scope:

- period pains and PMT
- headaches and migraines
- sluggish energy levels
- not feeling 'quite right'
- certain types of depression
- arthritis
- insomnia
- difficulties in conceiving
- chronic indecision
- stress in its many manifestations
- poor memory
- unclear thinking
- emotional disturbances.

The World Health Organisation (WHO) lists many conditions that acupuncture has been proved to treat effectively. These include:

- adverse reactions to radiotherapy and/or chemotherapy
- allergic rhinitis

- depression
- period pains
- facial pain
- headaches
- hypertension
- induction of labour
- knee pain
- lower back pain
- morning sickness
- nausea
- rheumatoid arthritis
- sciatica
- tennis elbow
- arthritis of the shoulder.

The WHO lists even more conditions where acupuncture has been shown to be effective but further proof is needed. These include:

- acne vulgaris
- alcohol dependence
- bronchial asthma
- female infertility
- fibromyalgia
- insomnia
- labour pain
- male sexual dysfunction
- drug dependence
- osteoarthritis
- polycystic ovary syndrome, etc.

There is a great deal of research currently taking place as to the effects of acupuncture and moxibustion therapy, some of which is being funded by the British Acupuncture Council. This, hopefully, will bring proof of the effectiveness of treating many more conditions than those listed above, which present-day practitioners know through their own experience, to be beneficial to the people in this 21st century.

To help select the correct points a number of diagnostic principles are used. One of these is the reading of the 12 Chinese pulses, six on each wrist, which relate to the ten organs and two functions. Each pulse gives the volume and quality of Qi present in each of the meridians and, from this, the practitioner can tell if there is too little, too much, or a blockage in them, (see previous chapter).

Some acupuncturists observe the colour and state of the tongue coating. Others, particularly those using the Law of the Five Elements as a guide, are more interested in the facial colour, voice tone, inappropriate emotion and one of the five odours exhibited by the patient. Other observations that can be taken into account are: the state of the nails, food cravings, favourite colour and season, bodily characteristics (physiognomy), information given from abdominal palpation, dreams, inappropriate heat distribution and childhood experiences.

These diagnostic signs, together with the information provided by the 12 pulses form the basis of treatment. Furthermore they can tell the trained practitioner where the problem lies, well before it develops into a more serious condition.

Because the twelve meridians run bilaterally, that is up or down both sides of the body, a test using a lighted taper is used to see if one side has more energy in it than the other. This test, mentioned previously, is called the Akabane test and the balancing of the weaker side is often one of the first treatments given.

Sometimes patients will get a reoccurrence of their symptoms which may last up to 48 hours. This is quite common and is considered positive as it follows the Law of Cure. This Law states that we get better from above to below, from the inside to the outside and in reverse chronological order.

Acupuncture was, and still is, effective as a preventive form of medicine and information on this is covered at length in the following chapter.

No system of medicine has ever had the answer to every illness because a human being is far more complex than we realise; what works for one doesn't always work for another. This quote from the *'Nei Jing'* presents this understanding well:

'Alas, medicine is so subtle that no one seems able to know its complete secrets. It's way is so wide that its scope is as immeasurable as the Heaven and the Earth, and its depth is as immeasurable as the four seas.'

However, many of us now are in the fortunate position to gain from the best of two worlds. On the one hand we have access to the wonders of modern Western Medicine with its powerful life-saving drug therapy, its surgical techniques which seem to improve year after year and its ability to treat acute and emergency conditions effectively. Furthermore it has at its disposal a formidable array of complex diagnostic techniques. On the other we have therapies from the Oriental Medical field of which Traditional Acupucture forms an important part. Here the focus is on the uniqueness of the individual and the enhancement of their restorative powers. Another of its strengths is in the treatment of chronic conditions which Western Medicine often struggles with; it is also effective as a preventive form of medicine so that we don't end up "digging a well when already weak from thirst". One of the biggest employers in the European Union, the UK's National Health Service, has also realised the importance of preventive medicine and has introduced certain measures for those of pensionable age where the physical aspects of the patient are monitored for any signs of a deterioration in health.

Thus a person is able to benefit, like never before, from treatments that address not only the body but their mental, emotional and spiritual aspects too which seems to me a very fortunate situation to be in.

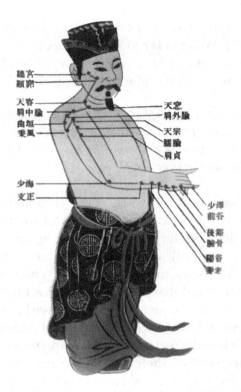

Figure 3   The Small Intestine Meridian

Preventive Medicine and Measures

Of all the systems of medicine available to us today whether it be genetic, Western orthodox, Oriental, alternative, Tibetan, ayurvedic, native American, shamanistic, vibrational or nutritional etc. the highest form has got to be preventive. This idea is not new; it goes back a long way to the time of the *Nei Jing* (c. 221 BCE) and is well encapsulated by this quote taken from it:

> *"To administer medicine for illnesses that have already developed, or to attempt to restore order only after unrest has broken out, it is as though someone has waited to dig a well after they have become weak from thirst; or those who start to forge weapons when the battle is already underway. Are these actions not too late?"*

Another quote, paraphrased, from an earlier text, the *Dao de Jing*, puts it this way:

> *"Before symptoms develop it's easy to take preventive measures,*
> *Deal with things in their formative state*
> *Put things in order before disorder sets in."*

In other words, "a stitch in time saves nine."

Around the time these early observations on the importance of preventive medicine were written, it is said that the physician was paid to keep the patient well — a concept similar to having one's car serviced. If the patient became ill, payment ceased and the practitioner would then have to bring the patient back to health, free of charge. Of course, the patient would have to follow closely the advice of the practitioner, who would, as now, recommend some lifestyle changes and regular seasonal treatment at the very least. Although there is uncertainty as to the source of this observation, in terms of a nation's health service, it must rank as one of the most effective ever in serving the needs of the people.

Health is the natural state of the universe and of its creation, humankind. Even if there are a few hiccups in this healthy state it is usually only temporary just as the seasons are sometimes erratic. Illness doesn't usually start overnight but often has its roots going back in time and commonly arises from long term lifestyle issues or chronic unresolved emotional stress or conflicts.

There is an enormous amount we ourselves can do to ensure that we don't get ill. At the root of it is rediscovering ways in which we can enhance and optimise, both internally and externally, our Qi energy so that longevity in good health can become a reality for us. The Chinese termed it "self-cultivation" or "nourishing life". This covers, on the one side, the strengthening and toning of the physical body through to the cultivation of our higher inner energies on the other.

One of the benefits of getting older is that we don't take things for granted quite so much as we did before. We know that each day is precious and in older age it's easier to appreciate this and not to waste it worrying about the past, what's going to happen in the future or what people may think of us. The emotions ease a bit too, not so much anger or lust; things become a bit more balanced of their own accord; feeling contented is a little bit more accessible and takes on a higher priority.

So in this chapter we will cover some aspects of the preventive measures we can take such as nutrition, exercise, acupuncture and moxibustion, Five Element healing music, lifestyle issues and feng shui all of which are ways which can "nourish life".

Nutrition — Eating and Drinking

So much has been written on nutrition, foods and diets to a degree that it all gets very confusing. However, common sense is one of the best ingredients to use. Remember — we want to do ourselves a favour by utilising the best and tastiest of fuels available to keep us functioning at our optimum best. To keep it simple it is recommended that 40–45% of our food intake should consist of vegetables and fruit, a similar percentage of grains and carbohydrates and the remainder 10–20% the richer foods such as meat, fish, eggs, dairy produce, fats, oils and sugar. For vegetarians and vegans it is even more important for them to use the highest quality foods available; what we eat and drink has an enormous bearing on our health — more than we realise.

Just as there are elemental associations with colours, flavours, emotions, seasons and musical notes etc. so there are with foods. Over the years practitioners, notably Leslie Cerier who wrote the *Quick and Easy Organic Gourmet* and Anne Marie Colbin, who wrote *The Natural Gourmet*, originally adapted from John Garvey's The Five Phases of Food: How to Begin (Wellbeing Books, 1983), have found that certain foods and their tastes and colours can support or strengthen each one of the five elemental forces. The following are a list of these particular foods. You may like to incorporate these into your daily diet — taking some from each section to create balance but also focussing on those that relate to the one Element within your system that is most in need of support. Over the years there have been different thoughts as to which category some foods belong. But use your intuition and taste buds and try to rotate each section sensibly bearing in mind which ones are in season. We touched upon some of these foods in the chapter on the Elements but here is a much more extensive list. It is divided into 13 categories which cover grains and tubers; dry beans and legumes; vegetables; fruits; seeds; herbs; nuts; dairy produce; seafood; fowl; meat; miscellaneous and cooking methods.

Foods that support the Wood Element:

Wood's flavour is sour which cools the body, cleanses the Liver and consolidates our energy. Leafy green vegetables all have an affinity with this Element:

Barley, oats, rye, wheat, spelt

Green lentils, mung beans, black eyed peas, split peas, peanuts

Globe artichoke, green pepper, broccoli, lettuce, parsley, green beans, green peas, rhubarb, summer squash

Apple (sour), cherry, avocado, coconut, grapefruit, kiwi, lemon, lime, sour orange, pineapple, plum, pomegranate

Alfalfa

Saffron, caraway, cumin, marjoram, bay leaf, dill, nutmeg, tarragon, cloves

Brazil nuts, cashew nuts

Egg yolk, mayonnaise, sour cream, sour yoghurt, butter

Trout and mackerel

Chicken

Fats, Liver (beef, lamb)

Nut butters, oils, olives, sour pickles, sauerkraut, vinegar, wheatbran, wheatgerm, wheatgrass, yeast

The recommended cooking method is shallow or stir frying which is a healthy way to preserve the goodness and flavours, particularly of vegetables.

Foods that support the Fire Element:

The bitter flavour corresponds to the Fire Element and can help regulate heat in the system. It penetrates to the Heart and the Small Intestine:

Amaranth, popcorn, quinoa, corn (yellow)

Red lentils

Asparagus, red pepper, broccoli, brussel sprouts, chicory, chives, collard greens, endive, kale, okra, scallions, swiss chard, turnip and tomato

Apricot , guava, kumquat, persimmon, raspberries, strawberries

Apricot kernels, sesame, sunflower

Hing (asafetida), hops

Pistachios, bitter almonds

Shrimp

Squab

Heart (beef), lamb

Beer, bitter coffee, chocolate, wine

The recommended method of cooking is roasting or grilling both of which help preserve the minerals and vitamins in the food and impart heat to the body.

Foods that support the Earth Element:

Earth's flavour is sweet which penetrates to the Stomach and the Spleen. In moderation they strengthen a deficiency but in excess can produce heat, damp or phlegm within the system so keep an eye on how you react to them:

Millet, sweet potato, yam

Chickpeas

Jerusalem artichoke, bamboo shoot, corn on the cob, eggplant (aubergine), kuzu (kudzu), mallow, parsnip, pumpkin, spagetti squash, winter squash, tapioca

Apples (sweet), banana, breadfruit, cantaloupe melon, cassava, coconut milk, sweet currants, dates, figs, sweet grapes, honey-dew melon, mango, mulberries, sweet orange, papaya, prunes, raisins, sweet cherries, tangerine

Pumpkin

Allspice, anise, cardamon, cinnamon, liqorice, turmeric, vanilla

Almonds, pecans, pine nuts, macademia nuts

Cottage cheese, ricotta cheese, ice cream, milk, sweet yoghurt

Fresh anchovies, salmon, swordfish, canned tuna

Pheasant, quail

Mutton, rabbit

Carob, honey, barleymalt, maple syrup, brown sugar, sweet chocolate

The recommended cooking method is boiling.

Foods that support the Metal Element:

The Metal Element manifests in food as the pungent flavour which stimulates the body and penetrates to the Lungs and Large Intestine:

Brown and white rice, sweet rice, potato

Navy beans, lima beans, soy beans, tempeh, tofu

Bok choy (white), cabbagae, capers, cauliflower, celeriac, celery, chilli, chinese cabbage, cress, cucumber, garlic, ginger, iceberg lettuce, kohlrabi, leeks, onions, radishes, rape, shallots, spinach, turnips, watercress, water chestnuts

Peach, pear

Dill

Basil, cayenne, coriander, fennel, fenugreek, mint, horseradish, black pepper, white pepper, thyme, sage

Hickory, walnut

Aged cheese, egg white

Cod, flounder, haddock, halibut, herring, perch

Turkey

Beef

The recommended cooking method is baking.

Foods that support the Water Element:

The salty flavour corresponds to Water and moves energy downwards and inwards. It penetrates to the Kidney and Bladder and regulates water metabolism within the system.

Buckwheat

Aduki beans, black soy beans, Kidney beans, pinto beans

Agar-agar, beets, burdock, dulse, Irish moss, kelp, kombu, mushrooms, nori, radicchio, red cabbage, salsify, wakame, water chestnuts

Blackberries, black raspberries, blueberries, boysenberries, concord grapes, cranberries, watermelon

Chia, black sesame

Chestnuts

Caviar, abalone, catfish, clam, crab, cuttlefish, lobster, mussels, octopus, oysters, sardines, scallop, squid

Duck

Ham, Kidney, pork

Decaffeinated coffee, sesame salt, miso, pickles (brine cured) seasalt, soy sauce (tamari), umeboshi plums, umeboshi vinegar, bancha tea.

The recommended cooking method is steaming which preserves the nutrients and maintains the flavours particularly of vegetables. If you add salt to your food keep it in moderation as an excess can have a detrimental effect on the Kidneys. Seasalt is best as table salt is refined and the good stuff, such as valuable minerals, is taken out.

Adapted and reprinted by kind permission from *The Quick and Easy Organic Gourmet* by Leslie Cerier (www.lesliecerier.com), Station Hill Openings Ltd., Barrytown, 1996.

Drinking

The same objective of keeping the system at its optimum best through foods also applies to what we drink. There are so many different types available but, of course, the best, and unfortunately the most boring, is plain water. It's worth remembering that 65–70% of our bodies are made up of it, but slowly dries up with age.

The reason why water is so good is that Nature, in the first place, has provided it for us, and in the second, it helps flush out and purify the system particularly the organs of the Kidneys and Liver. Although in the West the water companies have cleaned it it still can contain too many chemicals, especially chlorine, when it comes out of the tap. If it does, you can buy an inexpensive water filter to sort that out. It is recommended that we drink around 1½–2 litres of it a day. To counteract the blandness of it you might add lemon juice or alternatively, drink sparkling water: you will definitely notice the benefits if you persist. The other excellent drink, which has become popular in the West in recent years, is green tea containing as it does the Vitamins A, C and E and minerals especially selenium. It strengthens the immune system, helps prevent Heart disease, lowers cholesterol and slows down the ageing process.

Nutrition in Older Age

In our youth we can usually eat pretty much anything and get away with it. However as the years progress this is less easy to do and we need to adjust our diet accordingly.

Stomach acid and enzymes, which often decline in older age, have an important part to play in the absorption of nutrients from our foods. The mineral Zinc is one that needs to be kept at an optimal level because Stomach acid production partly depends on it. So ensure you get enough of this mineral (see the Wood Element section for suggestions on this) and if you suffer from digestive problems then digestive enzymes which, too, can aid in Stomach acid production, are worth considering.

Other vitamins and minerals that need to be kept at optimal levels, as they can be poorly absorbed, are Vitamin B12 and Folic Acid. Vitamin B12 can be found in foods such as salmon, sardines, chicken, lamb, beef, yoghurt and milk. Folic Acid (Vitamin B9) can be found in foods such as beans and legumes, green leafy vegetables, wheatgerm, potatoes and cauliflower etc. Furthermore some nutritionists suggest increasing our daily intake of Vitamin C and E as our age progresses. These can be found in many fruits, especially citrus, in lots of vegetables, and nuts and seeds (Vitamin E).

Another common cause of suffering in older age are aching joints and arthritis. As mentioned elsewhere in this book exercise, acupuncture or one of the manipulative therapies can often help with these conditions. However, for some people one of the causes can be certain foods that exacerbate these symptoms. The main culprits are acidic fruits, preservatives and colourings, cheese, red meats, alcohol and tomatoes (the latter have a high acid content). You might try and cut all of these out for five days and if the pain is coming from one or more of them you will usually notice an easing of symptoms within that time. The next stage is to reintroduce one food at a time and wait for three days before trying the next to see if the pain returns after this reintroduction; this will usually indicate the main culprit. Sometimes it is the one food we crave which can be the source of our discomfort. If it is to do with some of the foods or drinks you are consuming the result can be dramatic when you cut them out.

The incidence of Dementia and Alzheimer's Disease appears to be on the increase in this century. If the signs can be recognised early on you can take preventive measures to counteract them. These can include regular acupuncture treatment, certain nutritional supplements such as Vitamin C and E and Omega 3 (an essential fatty acid which is found in oily fish, blackcurrant seeds and walnuts). Vitamin B12 and B6 (found in meat, eggs, fish, poultry, brewers yeast, chickpeas and milk products) can also help to reduce the risk as they help in lowering levels of cortisol and homocysteine — the stress hormones. What is also thought to help is reducing our exposure to aluminium and mercury commonly found in cookware and dental amalgam fillings respectively. Information is just now coming to light of the benefits of Coconut Oil taken internally which may help to reverse some of the symptoms of both Dementia and Alzheimer's Disease. A very helpful book on this subject is *Alzheimer's Disease: What If There Was a Cure? The Story of Ketones* by Mary Newport, M.D. (Basic Health Publications Inc.)

Keeping the mental faculties active is another important measure that we should all try to incorporate into our daily lives if at all possible. These can include: doing crossword puzzles on a daily basis, playing bridge or chess, maintaining social conversations, keeping a pet, learning how to get better at the computer, learning another language, self-publishing a book or researching your family history etc.

Exercise

One of the most important factors that helps maintain our health throughout life, particularly as we get older, is keeping the body active and supple through daily exercise. It doesn't need to be too much or too complicated: briskly walking a mile or so a day will be worth its weight in gold. A Chinese text of some antiquity refers to the benefits of walking as it relaxes the muscles and tendons and strengthens the limbs whilst a more recent study in the US showed that women who walk for three hours a week were less prone to heart problems. A study of over 200 elderly people that was published in the Daily Telegraph in early 2013, showed that those who took a short walk at least four times a week had a 40% better survival rate than those who did not. Walking also activates six of the 12 main acupuncture meridians that flow throughout the body. These relate to the Bladder, Kidneys, Gallbladder, Liver, Stomach and Spleen. It also activates the only acupuncture point that is on the sole of the foot. This point relates to the Kidney energy and, whilst walking, helps draw energy from the earth up into the system. Here are some suggestions you might consider if you don't already have an exercise or fitness regime in place at the present time:

Yoga, Tai Qi and Qigong

These exercises or postures have all been developed and refined over a long period of time, some as far back as 200 BCE. The aim of them is twofold: firstly, they physically stretch, loosen and relax our muscles and ligaments which is essential as we get older, because that's when they tend to contract causing aches pains and stiffness; at the same time they help to tone the system, including the organs.

Secondly, they work like a form of meditation as they help to focus our attention within so that calmness and serenity can be experienced. The main obstacle to this daily practice is discipline as it takes effort, just like meditation, to do it. It's easily put off, to be replaced by all the other things in life we think we should be doing. You might benefit from joining a local group which will help with motivation and inspiration to keep you going. You will certainly benefit from this effort as it's all part of the preventive measures we can take in our daily lives to oil the wheels both physically and mentally. Chinese exercises, particularly, have been designed to focus on aligning our bones and joints, stretching and toning the ligaments and tendons and stimulating the circulation of Qi, blood, bile, lymph and other bodily fluids. Certain schools of Tai Qi and Qigong use the Law of the Five Elements in their regime which focus on supporting each Element and thus their associated organs or functions. Pilates or Ballroom Dancing are other methods that help stretch our muscles and ligaments. Most of the above are available in many towns and villages these days and the internet is probably the easiest way of locating a teacher or group although word of mouth is always the best source.

For those who live in bungalows, exercise is even more important because you are not using stairs and thus the leg muscles can become underused. This can lead to leg ulcers because the system has become sluggish. Keeping the legs raised whilst sitting can help prevent these occurring as it facilitates the circulation of blood just as exercise does.

Osteopathy, chiropractic, physiotherapy, or bowen technique are therapies that you may consider as these all help to keep the structure and consequently the muscular system in good order.

Our nutritional state can be assessed by non-invasive techniques such as kinesiology, hair analysis or a simple blood or saliva test. These can indicate which nutrients may be lacking within us — the main culprits being B12, Stomach acid, Magnesium, Vitamin C, Zinc etc. particularly as we get older.

Acupuncture and Moxibustion

Seasonal acupuncture treatment is considered important because it is in each season that a more potent effect can be had from using the correct points at the right time of year. This is because each Element resonates or has a strong affinity with a particular time of year the correspondences of which are shown in Diagram 2 (p. 10). By using the correct point in the correct season and, if possible, within the corresponding two-hour period, this treatment can 'brush the ash' off that particular meridian, allowing it to shine forth brightly or, in other words, bringing out its inherent potential to the fullest. Thus the Earth points are used on the Earth meridians (Stomach and Spleen) in the late summer, the Metal points on the Metal meridians (Lungs and Large Intestine) in the autumn and so on.

Seasonal treatment also allows patients, who rarely have the time, to look at their own life and health for a moment, which in itself can lead to helpful changes in outlook or lifestyle. All this helps in keeping our energies balanced and by doing so the seeds of disease, which are all around us on different levels, are kept from putting their roots down.

There are also a number of acupuncture points that can be used in older age to strengthen the immune system and help a person cope better with daily life. One of the most famous of these lies just below the knee. It is greatly effective for supporting the immune system, strengthening our defensive Qi, and is said to bestow longevity, endurance and helps keep us free from disease. It is the 36th point on the Stomach meridian and can be moxa'ed up to 20 times. Another point that lies on the arm is called "Nourishing the Old" and is a point that, when used with moxibustion, can help a person cope better with life as they get older. These points can both be effectively used at home with moxibustion provided your acupuncturist feels it is safe and appropriate and that you have thoroughly understood the process of applying it. Hopefully you and your family members, or house mates will be OK with the pungent aroma that moxa produces!

Music, Sound and the Five Elements

In most cultures of the world, music and sound have played a significant role in the ceremonial and cultural aspects of the nation. Whether in the ritualistic drumming of the African tribes, the specialised chanting of the Tibetan or Gregorian monks, the ancient music of the Australian Aborigines or the highly evolved representation of the inner harmonies as reflected in the sitar music of India, the effects have been extraordinarily profound.

A study conducted by the British Academy of Sound Therapy (BAST) found that 95% of clients suffering from stress felt an increased state of calm following sound treatment therapy. According to Dr Tomatis, the founder of Sound Therapy, our ears are connected to many other organs in our body by nerve paths, and so what we hear may contribute to the way they operate. In acupuncture terms the meridians of the Small Intestine, Three Heater and Gallbladder all pass through or near the ear and have a bearing on its function. The Kidney energy also has a connection to hearing and the ear. He also discovered that most of the sensory cells in the inner ear are accummulated in the high frequency zone. This suggests that our best response is to sounds above 8000 Hz and not the low frequency hum of chatter, traffic and computers which cause stress and fatigue.

In China music and sound have similarly played an integral part in that nation's culture from very ancient times being used in ritualistic ceremonies such as courtship and ancestral worship. It was believed able to connect the people with the spirits of their ancestors and the Emperors with the power of Heaven. Recently a number of seven hole flutes have been discovered there in a tomb calculated to be around 8,000 years old. In another, from 433 BCE, a complete orchestra was found containing zithers, flutes, drums, chime stones and 65 bells which can still be used today to play music composed on a five pitched scale. But it is the healing emphasis of a sector of this nation's music which sets it apart from those of other cultures. It focuses on maintaining health, lifting the spirits and as a healing vehicle which resonates with our inner selves particularly with regard to the Five Element system.

The skill of their musicians and composers was brought to a highly advanced state during the Han dynasty (221 BCE — 220 CE) when music became directed towards this therapeutic goal of achieving harmony between body mind and spirit. It was at the beginning of this dynasty that the *Nei Jing* was compiled which provided the theoretical foundation for the practice of all healing arts in China, including music. One of its main theories is the understanding that the internal nature of disease arises from disturbances in a person's emotional state. Thus too much anger, fear, grief, worry, over-excitement or sadness or conversely a lack of these, could disturb a person's health.

Today, in the developed countries of the world particularly in the West, it is these emotional imbalances which have become prevalent in society.

Chinese Five Element healing music has been found to help in therapeutically addressing them by bringing harmony to a patient's internal state.

Five different notes or tones (the pentatonic scale) were found to resonate with the five elemental forces in nature. By utilising and interweaving them together they help regulate the circulation of Qi energy within a person. This in turn was found to improve the functioning of the internal organs, balance the emotions, strengthen the psychological condition and stimulate the immune system.

Each Element has a corresponding note which is shown in Diagram 14 (p. 157) below:

This music is not composed of a single tone although it holds the central theme whilst surrounding it in an orderly way by other tones in a particular sequence or combination.

The Cheuh tone resonates with and regulates the Wood Element. It helps to release energetic blockages or the presence of excessive Qi within the associated organs of the Liver and

Element	Wood	Fire	Earth	Metal	Water
Note/ Tone	Chueh (F)	Chiah (G)	Kung (C)	Shang (D)	Yu (A)
Organ or Function	Liver/ GallBladder	Heart/ Small Intestine/ Heart Protector and Three Heater	Stomach and Spleen	Lungs/ Large Intestine	Bladder and Kidney
Emotion	Anger or lack of confidence	Joy or sadness	Worry or emotional rejection	Excess grief or lack of it	Excess fear or lack of it

Diagram 14

Gallbladder thus bringing about an ease of flow within them. It is particularly effective for those people who experience too much anger or irritability or conversely those who lack courage and determination in their lives.

The Chiah (aka Jyy) tone relates to the Fire Element and has the characteristics of growth, maturity and liveliness. Therapeutically it is recommended for vertigo, fatigue, muscular weakness and circulatory problems. Furthermore this music can benefit the Heart function and helps in situations where a person is suffering from conflicts in their personal relationships. This is because it also resonates with the Heart Protector and the Three Heater functions.

The Kung tone relates to the Earth Element which itself corresponds to the late summer. It helps promote a feeling of stability, groundedness and calmness within a person as it resonates with the Stomach and Spleen energies. It is therapeutically helpful for symptoms such as nausea, digestive disorders, insomnia and obsessive thinking.

The Shang tone influences the Metal Element and its associated organs, the Lungs and Large Intestine. The instruments traditionally used here are gongs and bells which can be effective in treating all types of respiratory disorders, the presence of excessive grief or where a person is stuck and feels unable to let go and move on in their life.

The Yu tone relates to the Water Element and to the winter. This type of music is traditionally played using two of the oldest musical instruments in China — the guqin and the guzheng. They are both "long zithers" and have been in existence prior to 433 BCE. This music helps the Qi to descend within a person and resonates with the Kidney energy. Therapeutically it is recommended for anxiety, disturbed sleep, asthma and problems associated with the Kidneys such as impotence, premature ejaculation and, particularly, excessive fear.

This Five Element healing music can be enjoyed at any time during the year but when listened to in the season that corresponds to each Element (see Diagram 2, p. 10) its effect becomes even more pronounced.

More information can be found on: www.Wind-Records.com

Lifestyle

Addictions

For those troubled with addictions to tobacco, recreational drugs or excessive consumption of alcohol, ear acupuncture and hypnotherapy can provide a means of successfully withdrawing from their grip. Addictions or obsessive compulsions can degrade the quality of our good Qi energy and take the sparkle out of life. Life coaching or counselling are other therapies you might consider as they can help bring focus and perspective which can then enable a person to make the right choices in their life.

Feng Shui

When it comes to unseen energy fields there are some people who experience them, some who don't but are open to the idea, and others who refute their existence. This is one of the reasons why some people dismiss the whole idea of acupuncture with its meridian system, acupoints and Qi energy. The concept of harnessing the energies flowing through the earth, which is the basis of Feng Shui, is also a difficult one to comprehend. There are people who, without doubt, feel or sense the presence of energies in manmade structures and in Nature — I don't personally but am open to the fact that others can. However I have witnessed divining rods (used for dowsing) being strongly agitated by these energies emanating from the earth, notably during one summer solstice near a stone circle on Ilkley Moor in Yorkshire.

Feng Shui, which is a system of geomancy thought to predate the origins of acupuncture, works with these subtle energies in the external environment. Originally it was used to identify a dwelling place where families could flourish in safety and also to determine the most auspicious burial sites for the dead. Nowadays it is used to regulate and optimise these energies within a person's living or working environment.

The aim is to figure out the best way in which the Qi in a home, garden or office can flow in the most harmonious and beneficial manner. To do this practitioners utilise specific compass directions relating to the layout of the home and harness the influence of certain colours, shapes and the position of objects within it. They may consider the family dynamics including date of birth and thus the astrological influences of those living there, the position of the surrounding buildings, the landscape and the proximity of water. All this information, and others depending on the style used, will help determine the solutions they will recommend so you might benefit the most in your living and working life. Many practitioners of Feng Shui incorporate the laws of Yin and Yang and the Five Elements in their practice. Thus the information from the questionnaires in the Chapter on the Elements, giving an indication of your elemental balance, will be of use to some of them.

Feng Shui cannot guarantee health, wealth or happiness but what it can do is optimise and enhance what we already have. In this regard it is similar to acupuncture which regulates and enhances the energies within a person whereas Feng Shui harmonises and optimises those in the external environment.

The Internet is again the most straightforward way of finding a qualified practitioner in your area.

Hearing and Eyesight

Our hearing, another of Nature's engineering wonders, is influenced by the function of the Kidneys which in turn are governed by the Water Element. Nowadays, with modern technology, our hearing can be greatly enhanced if it's starting to fail and modern aids can be programmed to enhance the hearing in each individual ear. Similarly with our eyesight, which is influenced by the Liver energy and governed by the Wood Element. The rapid advances in simple and safe laser therapy for repairing and even replacing lenses can allow us to keep our eyes in a good state for a lot longer than ever before. It is strongly advised, however, as a matter of course, that we have our eyesight checked every year. The equipment is very sophisticated these days and the ophthalmologist can easily check to see if there are any signs of degeneration at an early stage (such as glaucoma) when preventive treatment will have a much greater chance of working. An excellent hobby, incidentally, which keeps us active and which can be extremely helpful for our eyesight, is the game of table tennis.

Meditation

We all know that life is a gift which needs to be appreciated each day if possible and meditation can help unwrap it. It has the same root meaning as the word "medicine", referring to the core or centre of a person; its objective is to take our attention from the outside and place it on the inside, where peace and tranquillity reside. The philosopher Socrates alluded to this aspiration in his exhortation 'know thyself'.

There are many different types of meditation; some use a mantra or forms of chanting which is the repetition of a sacred word or words; others focus on the coming and going of the breath. Some use visualisation techniques which centre on areas of transformation in the body such as the *Dan Tian* (also called the Cinnabar Field), which lies about four fingers width below the belly button and which is one of the main areas of focus during Qi Gong exercises. Some people seek a living teacher to bring it alive, others look for guidance from books whilst yet others focus on the inner senses of sound, vision and taste.

Qianlong, a famous Emperor from the Qing dynasty, would meditate each morning so that his mind and spirit could be clear in order that he might deal with the day's running of the empire with clarity and compassion.

Having said all this, the practice is not easy. It sounds simple enough, but try focussing on only ten of your breaths without the mind or thinking process getting in the way and you'll see what I mean; there's a bit of a struggle here. It's when we make this inward journey that the inner conflicts seem to raise their heads and trouble us, but with determination that tranquil place within can still be found and experienced. It needs to be a daily effort, if possible, because each day we are given is different from the previous one and if we can be centred and at peace within we don't waste it so much.

Whatever method you find that works for you, the main point is that we should experience tranquillity and peace in our lives — it's a basic human necessity. Within lies a simple joy, common to all human beings and fortunately it's built in.

Sex

In the Fire Element section it was mentioned about the need to restrict the number of ejaculations for men in order not to deplete their energy. However, in the same text, the Handbook of the Simple Girl (written in the Sui Dynasty 581–618 CE), there is a section that recommends a minimum number in order to keep that part of the system ticking over and these are: at 20 years of age every four days; at 40 every 16 days; at 60 every 30 days.

Although they should only be considered as guidelines, the idea of preserving our energies to maintain good health into older age is as a result of experiences and observations learnt over many centuries. This is what lies behind these suggested restrictions. There appears to be no restriction when it comes to women who don't seem to be as energetically affected to the same degree as men.

Winter Sun

Those who live in the colder and damper countries such as northern Europe, might consider spending a few weeks in the warmer, dryer climes during the winter months. Even a short stay can make an enormous difference to those suffering from arthritic or respiratory conditions or those affected by the SAD syndrome. It can benefit a person's health for the remainder of the year. Accommodation costs in these warmer countries is often very competitive for longer stays at this time of year.

Conclusion

Longevity in good health, achieved by focusing on the preservation and enhancement of a person's Qi, was considered a high priority in ancient times. Today, as the importance of preventive medicine and measures find their renaissance once more in our modern culture that same goal, by the same means, can be attained by us too.

The Emperor (the Heart and its "shen"); the Kingdom (the human body); its Ministers (the organs); and each individual citizen within it (the cells) all function symbiotically together on the levels of the body, mind and spirit. What happens in one affects the others.

A final quote from the *"Nei Jing"* emphasises the dangers of inner conflict and stagnation but, more importantly, the benefits of keeping our consciousness clear and our spirits up:

> 'If the Emperor does not radiate virtue then those under him will be in danger which will cause the closing and blocking of the ways, finally stopping communication and the body will be seriously injured. From this the nurturing of life will sink into disaster.
>
> However if the Emperor radiates virtue those under him will be at peace. From this the nurturing of life will give longevity from generation to generation, and the empire will radiate with a great light.' (Larre and Rochat de la Vallée. 2003. p. 170.)

Bibliography

The Secret Treatise of the Spiritual Orchid. C. Larre and E. Rochat de La Vallee. Monkey Press, 2003. www.monkeypress.net

The Seven Emotions. Psychology and Health in Ancient China. C. Larre and E. Rochat de La Vallee. Monkey Press, 1996. www.monkeypress.net

Wu Xing. The 5 Elements in Chinese Classical Texts. E. Rochat de la Vallee. Monkey Press. www.monkeypress.net

Traditional Acupuncture. Volume 2. Traditional Diagnosis. J. R. Worsley. Billings and Sons Ltd., Worcester, UK.

The Yellow Emperor's Classic of Internal Medicine. Trans. by Ilza Veith. University of California Press, 1949.

China — A Portrait of the People, Place and Culture. Dorling Kindersley, 2007.

City of Heavenly Tranquillity. J. Becker. Penguin Books.

The Forbidden City. G. R. Barme. Profile Books.

Forbidden City. The Great Within. Holdsworth and Courtauld. Frances Lincoln Limited.

The Acupuncture Handbook. Angela Hicks. Piatkus, 2006.

Acupuncture for Body, Mind and Spirit. Peter Mole. Spring Hill Books, 2007.

The China Study Tour. Compiled by Stuart Lightbody. Privately published, 1984.

The Qin Dynasty Terra-Cotta Army of Dreams. Xi'an Press, 2005.

Imperial China. Charis Chan. Penguin Books.

The Heart of the Dragon. Alisdair Clayre. Dragon Book ApS.

The Quick and Easy Organic Gourmet. Leslie Cerier. Station Hill Openings, Ltd. Barrytown, 1996.

Managing Pain and Other Medically Proven Uses of Acupuncture. Dr. R. Halvorsen. Gibson Square.

A Short History of Nearly Everything. Bill Bryson. Doubleday.

The Handbook of Five Element Practice. Nora Franglen. School of Five Element Acupuncture, 2004.

In the Footsteps of the Yellow Emperor. Peter Eckman, MD. Long River Press, San Francisco, 2007.

Further Reading:

Acupuncture for Body, Mind and Spirit. Peter Mole. Spring Hill Books, 2007.

A Simple Guide to Acupuncture: The Five Elements. Nora Franglen. SOFEA.

Between Heaven and Earth. Harriet Beinfeld and Efrem Korngold. Ballantine Books, 1991.

Appendix: Overseas Acupuncture Organisations

Some of the contact details in this document may be out of date. For up to date contact details, please go to http://www.icmart. org/members.html

Pan European organisation for European acupuncture associations:

PEFOTS
Geldersekade 87 A
1011 EK Amsterdam
The Netherlands
Tel/Fax: +31 (0)20 421 12861
Email: info@pefots.com
www.pefots.com

AUSTRALIA

Australian Acupuncture & Chinese Medicine Association
PO Box 5142
West End
Queensland 4101
Tel: +61 (0)7 3846 5866
Email: aacma@acupuncture.org.au
www.acupuncture.org.au

Australian Traditional Medicine Society
PO Box 1027
Meadowbank
New South Wales 2114
Tel: +61 (0)2 9809 6800
Fax: +61 (0)2 9809 7570
Email: info@atms.com.au
www.atms.com.au

Acupuncture Association of Victoria
126 Union Road
Surrey Hills, Victoria 3127
Tel: +61 1800 025 334

AUSTRIA

Österreichische Gesellschaft für Akupunktur (ÖGA)
Kaiserin Elisabeth Spital
Huglgasse 1-3
A-1150 Wien
Tel: +43 1 98104 5758
Fax: +43 1 98104 5759
Email: aku@kes.magwien.gv.at
www.akupunktur.at

Austrian Association of Acupuncture
President: Prof. Dr. Helmut Nissel
Schlosshoferstrasse 49
1210 Vienna
Fax: +43 1 278 72 72 7
Email: helmut.nissel@akupunktur.at

Austrian Medical Society for Neuraltherapy
Mrs Simone Paumann
Bahnhofbichl 13
6391 Fieberbrunn
Tel: +43 5354 52120

Fax: +43 5354 5300-731
Email: oenr@tirol.com
www.neuraltherapie.at

AZERBAIJAN

Azerbaycan National Acupuncture Association
President: Dr. Ehtibar Kazimov
Moskova Cad. N°82/1
Baku
Tel: 9941 2 66 98 77
Fax: 99412 47 98 78
Email: inam_med@mail.az

BELGIUM

Belgian Association of Medical Acupuncturists
President: Dr. Gilbert Lambrechts
Everselstraat 11
3580 Beringen
Tel: +32 11 42 44 80
Email: bvga@skynet.be
www.acupunctuur.be/

BRAZIL

Sociedade Medica Brasileira de Acupuntura — SMBA
Rua Almirante Lamego 1380
Florianopolis SC 88015-601
Tel: 048-972 1174
Fax: 048-222 5237
Email: smba@cfh.ufsc.br

A.B.A.-Brazilian Association of Acupuncture
R. Guarara,
242 - J. Paulista
São Paulo
Tel: 11-885 0524
Email: orley.dulcetti@mandic.com.br

Dr. Marcus Vinicius Ferreira M.D.
Rua Visconde de Piraja 414 sala 702
22410–002 Ipanema, Rio de Janeiro
Tel: 021 247 2480
Email: vinifer@ibm.net

BULGARIA

Bulgarian Association of Acupuncture
PO Box 33
1463 Sofia

BELORUSSIA

Acupuncture Association Byelorussian
Ministry of Health
Masherova Street, 47/1–170
220035 Minsk

CANADA

General information on acupuncture regulation, etc in Canada:
http://www.medicinechinese.com

The Canadian Acupuncture Foundation (Physios)
Suite 302
7321 Victoria Park Avenue

Markham
Ontario L3R 278

Chinese Medicine and Acupuncture Association of Canada
154 Wellington Street
London, Ontario N6B 2K8
Tel: 001 519 642 1970
Fax: 001 519 642 2932
Email: icma@webgate.net

Acupuncture Canada
742 King Street West
Suite #5
Kitchener, Ontario N2G 1E7
Tel: 001 519 579 2147
Email: info@acupuncture.ca
www.acupuncture.ca/contact.htm

Ordre D'Acupunctureus Du Quebec
1001 Boulvard D'Masonneauve
Bureau 403
Montreal
Quebec H2L 4P9
Tel: 001 514 523 2882
Fax: 001 514 523 9669
Email: info@ordredesacupuncteurs.qc.ca

CHINA

China Association of Zhenju
No 18 Beixincang China Dongzhimen
Beijing 100700

CROATIA

Croatian Medical Acupuncture Association
Krajiska 16/IV
41000 Zagreb

CYPRUS

Pancyprian Medical Society of Acupuncture
57 Aeschylos Street,
Nicosia

CZECH REPUBLIC

Czech Medical Society of Acupuncture
Sladkvskeho 657
530 02 Pardubice

Czech Medical Academy for Acupuncture and
     Complementary Medicine
Fuegnerova 35
613 00 Brno

DENMARK

Dansk Selskab for Akupunktur
Gammel Kongevej 80
1850 Frederiksberg C
Tel: 0045 31 212112

Danish Medical Association of Acupuncture
Nellikevej i
6400 Sonderborg

ICMART
GI. Kongevej 80
1850 Frederiksberg C

ESTONIA

Estonian Association of Acupuncture and Traditional
    Chinese Medicine
Voru 11
Tallinn
EEOO 10

FINLAND

The National Research and Development Centre for Welfare
    and Health
Silstasaaren 18A
PO Box 220
00531 Helsinki
Tel: 00358 900 531

Finnish Medical Acupuncture Society
Punakorvaantie 10
24800 Halikko

FRANCE

Association Française D'Acupuncture
3, avenue de l'Arrivée
75749 PARIS Cedex 15
Tel: 01 43 20 26 26
Fax: 01 43 20 54 46
www.acupuncture-france.com

Fédération National de Médicine Traditionelle Chinoise
7, rue Louis Prével
06000 Nice
Tel: +33 (0) 870 304 870
Fax: +33 (0) 4 93 82 31 39
www.fnmtc.com

Association de Formation Medicale Continue et de Recherche pour
le Diplome d'Acupuncture de l'Ouest
Chemin du Bois Durand
85300 Soullans

Societé d'Acupuncture d'Aquitaine
4, rue de Fleurus
33000 Bordeaux

GERMANY

Deutsche Ärztegesellschaft für Akupunktur (DÄGfA)
Würmtalstr. 54
81375 München
Tel: +49 (0)89 7 10 05-11
Fax: +49 (0)89 7 10 05-25

German Research Institute of Chinese Medicine
Silberbachstrasse 10
79100 Freiburg im Breisgau

Deutsche Gesellschaft für Akupunktur und Neuraltherapie (DGfAN)
(German Society for Acupuncture and Neuraltherapy)
Mühlweg 11
07368 Ebersdorf
Tel: +49 (0)3 66 51 5 50 75
Fax: +49 (0)3 66 51 5 50 74

Arbeitsgemeinschaft fuer klassische Akupunktur & Traditionelle
Chinesische Medizin e.v
Drakestr. 40

12205 Berlin
Tel: +49 30 84309650
Fax: +49 30 84309649
Email: noll@agtcm.de
www.agtcm.de

GREECE

Panhellenic Medical Acupuncture Society
34 Solonos Street
10673 Athens
Tel: +30 1 3637064
Fax: +30 1 6004707

Medical Acupuncture Association of Northern Greece
Dim. Gounari 4
54621 Thessaloniki
Greece
Tel: +30 31 239955
Fax: +30 31 234450
Email: karanik@med.auth.gr and alexlio@spark.net.gr

HUNGARY

Magyar Orvosi Kamara
1063 Budapest
Szinyei Merse Pal u.4
Tel: 00361 269 4391

Hungarian Medical Acupuncture Association
9021 Gyor
Bajcsy-Zs u.I

INDIA

Council of Alternative Systems of Medicines
3 Canal Street
Calcutta 700 014
Tel: 91-33-4718394/2465037
Fax: 91-33-4712164

Acupuncture Association of India (AAI)
188/87 Prince Anwar Shah Road
Calcutta–700 045
Tel: 033 4735778

IRELAND

Acupuncture Council of Ireland (TCMCI)
Station House
Shankhill
Dublin 18
Tel: +353 (0)1 2393267
www.tcmci.ie

ISRAEL

The Medical Society of Acupuncture of the Israeli Medical
     Association (MSAIMA)
32 Mahrazet Street
PO Box 3167
Bat-Yam 59 131

The Israel Association of Medical Acupuncture
4 Asher Levin Street
PO Box 260
Rishon-Le-Zion

Mr. Ron Samra
46/1 Nahal Zohar
Modiin 71700
Fax: 010 97236188932
(Set up the Israeli Council for Trad. Chin. Med. in Jan 1998)

ITALY

Associazione Medica Italiana di Agopuntura Didactica
P. Navona 49
00816 Roma
Tel: +39 6 6868556

Italian Society for Reflexology, Acupuncture and Auriculotherapy
Via G. Dandini 19
00154 Rome

Italian Medical Association of Acupuncture (AMIA)
Piazza Navona 49
00186 Rome

Italian Association of Manual Medicine and Neuroreflexotherapy
    (AIMAR)
Via Emiha Est, 18/1
41100 Modena

Research Institute of Clinical Homeopathy, Acupuncture
    and Psychotherapy
Via Sabotino 2
00195 Roma

INARM — Intern. Network for Acupuncture Research Methodology
Istituto Paracelso
Via Ippolito Nievo
61-00153 Rome
Tel: +39 6 5897364
Fax: +39 6 5816348

Italian Assoc. of Acupuncture-moxibustion & Trad.
   Chinese Medicine
Via Oreste Regnoli 8
00152 Rome
Tel: +39 6 5806459
Fax: +39 6 5816348

JAPAN

Japan Acupuncture Moxibustion and Ryoraku Medical Society
Karita 8-15-15
Sumiyoshi-ku
Osaka 558

Acupuncture Section of Japanese Society of Ryodoraku Medicine
1-10-15 Chuodori
Nichinan
Miyazaki 887

Japan Society of Acupuncture
3-44-14 Minami Otsuka Toshima-Ku
Tokyo 170-0005
Tel: 81-3-3985 6188
Fax: 81-3-3985-6188
Email: tsutani.cph@mri.tmd.ac.jp
www.lifence.ac.jp/acp_tokyo/index.htm

Japan Society for Oriental Medicine
Nakadori Bldg
2-2-20 Nihonbashi
Chuo-ku
Tokyo 103–0027
Tel: 81-3-3274 5060
Fax: 81-3-3274 4795
http://megacitynetwork.who.or.jp/Tokyo/Association/W-5ca

KOREA

Korea Acupuncture-Moxibustion Association
2F. #275-3 Sukchon-Dong,
Songpa-Gu
Seoul
Tel: 82-2-425 4437/8
Fax: 82-2-425–4439

LATVIA

Full Name: Latvian Medical Society
Association of Acupuiicture and Related Techniques
Dzirnavu str. 6-8
226000 Riga-10

LITHUANIA

Lithuanian Medical Doctors Association of Acupuncture and
   Traditional Medicine
Postfach 233 007,
Akademieklinik,
Kaunas

LUXEMBURG

Luxemburg Medical Association of Acupuncture
Rue Origer 5
L-2269 Luxemburg

NETHERLANDS

NTAV
Schiedamseweg 92a
3025AG Rotterdam
Tel: +31 476 3848

Zhong
Dutch Association for Traditional Chinese Medicine
Agro Businesspark 70
6708 PW Wageningen
Tel: 0317 479 740
info@zhong.nl
www.zhong.nl

Dutch Acupuncture Association
Van Persijnstraat 15-17
3811 LS Amersfoort
Tel: +31 33 4630434

Dutch Medical Acupuncture Association
Lytse Wijngaarden 8
8404 BA Langezwang

Nederlandse Artsen Acupunctuur Vereniging
Secretariaat
Postbus 8547
3503 RM Utrecht
Tel: +31 30-2474630
Fax: +31 30-2474439
Email: secretariaat@naav.nl
www.acupunctuur.com

NEW ZEALAND

New Zealand Register of Acupuncture
PO Box 9950

Wellington 1
Tel: +64 4 801 6400
www.acupuncture.org.nz

NORWAY

Norsk Forening for Klassik Akupunktur
Munchsgate 7
N-0165 Oslo
Tel: +47 22 36 17 74

Norwegian Medical Association of Acupuncture
3145 Tjome

Norwegian University of Traditional Chinese Medicine and
Acupuncture (NUKNA)
Parkvn. 51B
N-0256 Oslo
Tel: +47 22 563980
Fax: +47 22 563973
Email: nukna@communique.no
www.communique.no/NUKNA/

POLAND

Polskie Towarzystwo Akupunktury
ul. Winnicka 10
02–093 Warzawa
Tel: +48 22 659 8323
Email: PTAku@pharmanet.com.pl

Reflexotherapy Secition of Polish Medical Association
ul. Boya 6, m 57
00-621 Warsaw

PORTUGAL

Associação Portuguesa de Acupunctura
Rua Viriato, 27 3º A
Lisboa 1050–234
Tel: +351 21359 0474/5
Fax: +351 21315 2269
Email: apa-da@mail.telepac.pt

ROMANIA

Romanian Association of Alternative Medicine "Transylvania"
St. Progresului nr. 17
PO Box 35
4800 Baia Mare

RUSSIA

Russian Association of Acupuncture and Traditional Medicine
Vavilovich Street 14
195267 Saint Petersburg

SINGAPORE

Singapore High Commission
Director of Traditional Chinese Medicine
Ministry of Health
College of Medicine Building
16 College Road
Singapore 169854
Tel: 0065 223 7777

SLOVAKIA

Slovak Medical Society of Acupuncture
Clinic of Pneumology and TB
Podunajske Biskupice
825 56 Bratislava

SLOVENIA

Association of Acupuncture and Traditional Medicine of Slovenian
    Medical Society
Polanskova 3,
PP30, 61231 Ljubjiana

SOUTH AFRICA

Chiropractic Homeopathic and Allied Health Services
PO Box 17005
Groenkloof

The International Institute of Chinese Medicine & Acupuncture
PO Box 2246
19 Av. Disandt-Fresnaye
Cape Town 8000
Tel: 27-21-4341654

SPAIN

Practitioners Register
Fundacion Europa de Medicina Tradicional China
Av. de Madrid, 168 -170, Entlo A
Barcelona 08028

Tel: +34 902 16 09 42
Fax: +34 933 39 52 66
Email: mtc@mtc.com and pr@mtc.es
www.mtc.es

SRI LANKA

Ayurveda Medical Council
Dr. N.M. Perera Mawatha
Colombo 8
Tel: 00941 697437

The Register Open International University for Complimentary
    Medicines
28 International Buddhist Centre Road
Colombo 6
Tel: 94-1-585242
Fax: 94-1-584148/583337

SWITZERLAND

Assoziation Schweizer Ärztegesellschaften für Akupunktur und
    chinesische Medizin (ASA)
http://www.akupunktur-tcm.ch/

Schweizerische Ärztegesellschaft für Akupunktur — Chinesische
    Medizin (SAGA-TCM)
Postfach 2003
8021 Zürich

Schweizerische Ärztegesellschaft für Aurikulomedizin und
    Akupunktur (SÄGAA)
Postfach 176
8575 Bürglen
Tel: 071 634 66 19
Fax: 071 634 66 18

Ärztegesellschaft für Traditionelle Chinesische Medizin (AG-TCM)

Dr. med. Doris Lei
Wilfriedstrasse 8
8032 Zürich
Tel: 043 267 30 20
Fax: 043 267 30 25
Email: doris.lei@bluewin.ch

Dr. med. Doris Renfer-Martin
Kirchplatz 3
8953 Dietikon
Tel: 01 740 52 23
Fax: 01 740 48 45
Email: drenfer@smile.ch

Association Genevoise des Médecins Acupuncteurs (AGMA)
7, rue Hugo-de-Senger
CH-1205 Geneve
www.akupunktur-tcm.ch/agma

TURKEY

Turkish Acupuncture Association
Rumeli Cad. Efe Sk. 18/2
Osmanbey
Istanbul

USA

Council of Colleges of Acupuncture and Oriental Medicine
1424 16th Street NW, Suite 501
Washington, DC 20036

National Acupuncture and Oriental Medicine Alliance
1833 North 105th Street
Seattle, WA 98133

National Commission for the Certification of Acupuncturists
(NCCAOM)
11 Canal Center Plaza
Suite 300
Alexandria, VA 22314
Tel: 001 703 548 9004

American Association of Oriental Medicine
433 Front St
Catasauqua, PA 18032
Tel: 610-266 1433
Fax: 610-2768
www.aaom.org/states.html

Index

Printed in the United States
By Bookmasters